REAL MEN DO YOGA

REAL MEN

— DO —

YOGA

21 Star Athletes Reveal Their Secrets
for Strength, Flexibility
and Peak Performance

John Capouya

Health Communications, Inc.
Deerfield Beach, Florida

www.hcibooks.com

Disclaimer

Yoga is fundamentally a very safe exercise, but it is also a challenging workout. As with any exercise program, check with your doctor before beginning your practice. And if you are in acute pain from an injury or experiencing a flare-up of back problems, allow yourself time to heal before starting. Yoga shouldn't hurt—if it does, ease up and/or stop exercising immediately. Don't force yourself into the positions and don't expect to emulate our yoga model, Glen, right off the bat; these stretches take time and patience to master.

Library of Congress Cataloging-in-Publication Data

Capouya, John, 1956–
    Real men do yoga : 21 star athletes reveal their secrets for strength, flexibility and peak performance / John Capouya.
        p. cm.
    Includes bibliographical references.
    ISBN-13: 978-0-7573-0112-4
    ISBN-10: 0-7573-0112-6
    1. Yoga, Haòha. 2. Exercise for men. I. Title.

RA781.7.C355 2003
613.7'046—dc21

2003051102

Publisher: Health Communications, Inc.
        3201 S.W. 15th Street
        Deerfield Beach, Florida 33442-8190

R-11-06

Cover design by Larissa Hise Henoch
Cover photo of Eddie George by Rob Lindsay
Collaborator and yoga consultant: Michael Lechonczak
Yoga photography by Erica Berger
Yoga model: Glen de Vries
Author photo by Suzanne Williamson
Inside book design by Dawn Von Strolley Grove

To Suzanne, beautiful in yoga and beyond.

To Dave, who brought me to yoga.

To Hugo, who taught me meditation.

To Eric, who gave me the idea for this book.

Contents

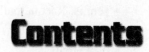

Acknowledgments

F irst I'd like to thank Michael Lechonczak, my collaborator and consultant on this book. Not only for his invaluable yoga insights and expertise, but also for the encouragement he gave me and the enthusiasm he brought to the project.

Hilary Lindsay, who teaches yoga in Nashville, Tennessee (see *activeyoga.com*), was incredibly generous and helpful. She knows yoga should be fun, and the folks in Nashville and I are lucky to have it that way.

Much appreciation to Paul Frediani, New York–based trainer and flexibility expert, for freely sharing his time, knowledge and contacts.

Eddie George, one of the first and most accomplished pro athletes to take up yoga, is also one of the most thoughtful and articulate. Thanks so much for being a part of this project, including posing for the cover picture.

Thanks to my agents, Nina Collins and David McCormick, for their counsel and support.

I'm grateful to the Dharma Yoga Center in New York City, where this addict gets his fix. They have the good stuff.

I'm also very thankful to yoga instructors around the country who gave their time and shared their experiences, including:

Alan Jaeger, who teaches yoga to pro baseball players at the Jaeger Sports Academy in Woodland Hills, California. His enthusiasm is contagious, and several of his prominent alumni are interviewed in this book.

Dr. Craig Aaron, who, with his wife, Jennifer Aaron, teaches Extreme Yoga for the Warrior Athlete in Atlanta.

Danny Poole ("Yoga Danny") in Denver; Charles DeFay of Synergy Yoga in Encinitas, California; Eric Paskel, owner and teacher at Sanga Yoga in the Detroit area; Katherine Roberts of Yoga for Golfers, based in Colorado; Sarah Pryor, who works with golfers and other athletes in Orlando; Jennifer Greenhut in L.A.; Nancy Nielsen in Denver; Sarah Margolis at New York's Yoga Connection; Eben Dennis in Plano, Texas; Annette Lang, flexibility expert and trainer in Brooklyn, New York; and Richard Allon of the Rasa Yoga Center in Manhattan, New York.

This book wouldn't have been possible without the pro athletes who told their yoga stories, starting with Eddie George. Joining him on the All-Yoga, All-Interview team (in no particular order): Sean Burke, Barry Zito, Kevin Garnett, Amani Toomer, Al Leiter, Steve Reed, Shannon Sharpe, J. L. Lewis, Mike Lieberthal, Lional Dalton, Diamond Dallas Page, Justin Gimelstob, Wally Sczcerbiak, Jack Krawczek, Tanner Eriksen, Dean Goldfine, Rod Smith, Robby Ginepri, Eric Hiljus, Kerry Kittles and Keith Washington.

Real thanks to all the Real Men who were interviewed. Your fellow men, starting with this one, really appreciate it. You are: David Cooke, Nick Cardillicchio, Tommy Bernard, Ken Canfield, Dan Levitan, Jerry Grossman, Peter Scirios, Jonathan Kelley, Ted Roman, G. W. Struz, Marty Stein, Mark Massara, Carey Bolton, Andy O'Keefe, Michael Flynn, Craig Bromberg, Bob Eriksen and Dave Herndon.

Thanks also to the sports coaches who talked to me about yoga and elite athletes, including Steve Watterson of the Tennessee Titans; Paul Hewitt (basketball) and Kenny Thorne (tennis) of Georgia Tech; Troy Wenzel of the Milwaukee Bucks; Jim Gillen and Steve Hess of the Denver Nuggets.

To all the sports reporters around the country who helped with this book: Great job. They include Luis Fernando Llosa, Pete Williams, Lynn DeBruin, Jon Rizzi, Mike Wells, Ohm Youngmisuk, Bob McManaman, Sarah Lorge Butler, Tom Keegan, Ryan Malkin and Gregg Goldstein.

Nancy Smith, your shrewd advice and encouragement meant a lot. Can't wait to read yours.

John Leland, Jerry Adler, Eric Messinger, Dave Herndon and David Friedman gave me great reads and editorial suggestions.

On the photo front: Kudos to Rob Lindsay for his cover and inside photography, plus extracurricular assistance and amiability.

Thanks to Erica Berger and John Engstrom for the great yoga photography.

And to Glen de Vries, our yoga model: looking good.

Suzanne Williamson's photo editing eye was sharp as always, and much appreciated.

The folks at *Yoga Journal,* in addition to putting out a great magazine, have been open, receptive and helpful, including Nora Isaacs, Matthew Solan, Guiv Rahbar and Dayna Macy. Namasté.

If I've overlooked anyone, I sincerely apologize. (Gotta meditate more and achieve greater clarity.)

Introduction:
Real Men Do Yoga

N o, you won't have to stand on your head. There will be no strange and painful contortions here.

No chanting, no incense, no gurus.

And, no, it isn't a chick thing.

These are probably the biggest misconceptions that some men still have about yoga. In the last few years, yoga has exploded in popularity in this country—some 15 million people do it. But because so many women practice yoga, and it's had a "fringe" or New Age image, lots of guys haven't tried yoga yet, and they think it really isn't for them.

Wrong! You see, none of these stereotypes need apply. Doing yoga doesn't require freak-show flexibility. Yoga's not some weird Eastern religion. In fact, it's not a religion at all. And—let me say this again—it's not just practiced by women. There are roughly 3.5 million men in the United States doing yoga right now, including some of the top athletes in professional sports.

So what is yoga, then?

At its heart, yoga is an amazing exercise system with 5,000 years of road-testing behind it. That long history, a growing body of medical evidence and the reports of men practicing yoga right now all tell us this: If you're a guy who wants to get in great shape—maybe the best shape of your life—yoga is the workout for you. It's fun, it's different, and it's a terrific complement to any other activities you currently enjoy.

This simple but incredibly effective method:

- *vastly improves flexibility*
- *increases strength and muscle tone*
- *instills superior balance and body control*
- *improves breathing and oxygen intake*

Since these are all essential qualities for sports, yoga also:

- *improves athletic performance*

That's why so many of America's top pro athletes are doing yoga, and why they were among the first American men to get with the program. In this book you'll hear directly from more than twenty of these sports stars—the guys you see on TV every Sunday. They'll tell you how yoga's taken their skills to a higher level and prolonged their careers. And you'll see some of these great athletes doing yoga, including legendary quarterback Dan Marino—turns out he was a yoga jock, too!

Here's a quick taste of the rave reviews athletes are giving yoga:

Eddie George, star NFL running back, Heisman Trophy winner: "Yoga's helped me to avoid injuries and made me stronger, particularly in the upper body. It gives me a competitive edge." (That's Eddie and his impressive upper body on the cover of this book.)

Barry Zito, pitcher, Cy Young Award winner: "It's helped me tremendously flexibility-wise, and the relaxation techniques calm me down, which is particularly important on the mound."

Kevin Garnett, NBA superstar: "I've been doing yoga since 1995, when I first came into the league, and I practice my breathing exercises before every game."

Sean Burke, All-Star NHL goaltender: "In sports, you need balance, strength and flexibility, and yoga helps so much in each of these areas. I truly believe that yoga has been a huge part of my success."

Today, yoga's all over the sports world. It's huge in golf: **David Duval** does a thirty-minute yoga workout every day. **Justin**

Gimelstob, a top-ranked tennis player who was having severe back problems, tells us in chapter 10 that "Yoga saved my career."

Sounds pretty good, right? But wait, as they say in the TV commercials, there's much, much more! Yoga also:

- *Prevents injuries and speeds up recovery*
- *Alleviates back pain*
- *Raises your energy level*
- *Recharges your sex life*
- *Gives you the best sleep of your life*

And those are just the physical benefits. The way yoga gets you to listen to your body—it's been described as a kind of meditation in motion—also hones your mental game, your approach to sports, work and your family life. As **Mike Lieberthal,** the All-Star catcher for the Philadelphia Phillies, says, "Yoga's as good for the mind as it is for the body." That's because it:

- *Reduces stress and minimizes its harmful effects on the body*
- *Relaxes you mentally as well as physically*
- *Trains your focus and concentration so you can perform at your peak—in The Zone*

Put all of the above together and it creates another huge upside to yoga that I haven't even mentioned yet—and it's one of the biggest payoffs of all.

- *Yoga just makes you feel great!*

Throughout this book, I'll explain how this ingenious exercise system works, laying out the physiology of it, citing studies and other medical evidence. But I don't think anyone has a complete scientific explanation for the overall feeling of well-being you get after a yoga workout—call it the yoga glow.

Jerry Grossman, a 43-year-old technical consultant who lives in New York City, says that his first class four years ago "had a magical effect on me, it was so reviving. It was the day after I had played some hoops and I was sore, but afterward I was a new man. For a day or so after I felt like a million bucks, but I wasn't really clued in yet to what was happening. Then I realized: 'It's the yoga.'"

As Jerry's example shows, it's not just pro athletes who have gotten wise to the wisdom of yoga. In this book you'll hear from men of all ages, all over the country, who've made yoga part of their lives. Here's the thing: These are not just the guys whom the stereotypes tell us do yoga. You know, sensitive New Age guys looking for enlightenment. Far from it.

In my research for this book, I've talked to, among others, firemen, architects, contractors, real estate developers, journalists, lawyers, restaurant owners, entrepreneurs, a truck driver in Nebraska and a bass player with the Detroit Symphony Orchestra. All they have in common is yoga. That's the point, as well as the title, of this book: Real Men Do Yoga.

Same as the pro athletes, these guys will tell you how yoga's gotten them in fantastic shape, taken away their back pain—and improved their golf! Some of these men laughingly call themselves yoga addicts, and swear they'll practice it for the rest of their lives. That's another yoga advantage: You're never too old to do it, enjoy it and benefit from it.

More good news: You can start to see all these results in just two hours a week. In this book I'll teach you how, coaching you through the yoga stretches one at a time, with easy-to-follow instructions and how-to pictures. We'll learn which positions are the best at producing each of yoga's many benefits: flexibility, strength, balance, etc.

Chapter 9 tells you how to prevent injuries with yoga and in chapter 11 you'll see which exercises help prepare you to excel in different sports, starting with golf. After all the physical moves, we'll get into yoga's mental benefits—better focus and relaxation—and learn how to meditate.

Then at the end of the book we put it all together in two routines: a

30-minute workout for beginners or rookies and a 45-minute workout
for veterans (that's you, once you've been practicing for a few
months). Michael Lechonczak, an absolutely superb yoga teacher in
New York City, helped me with the instruction. He's trained in
Ashtanga, Iyengar and Anusara yoga, all of which are derived from
the Hatha yoga tradition, and he's been teaching for ten years. Best of
all, Michael, who's a big, muscular guy himself, has put together yoga
workouts specially designed with mens' bodies—and our sometimes
macho attitudes—in mind.

Now consider this: Yoga's basically free. After you plunk down a
few bucks for this book and buy a mat to work out on (I'll tell you
what you need in the next chapter), yoga is available to you gratis, any
time you want it. You don't need any fancy equipment, so you can do
yoga anywhere, including in a hotel room on the road, which is great
for business travelers.

We've already demolished the idea that yoga is a chick thing. As
for yoga being a spiritual thing, that's entirely up to you. Some students and many teachers want to emphasize yoga's more metaphysi-
cal and spiritual aspects. And that's fine, if that's what you're after.

But we're just going to keep the focus on yoga's fantastic physical
and mental benefits, without getting into the more cosmic stuff. So
we'll be learning a twenty-first-century American kind of yoga, one
that's fun, results-oriented and practical. The way men like things.
That's the kind of yoga Tommy Bernard, a 55-year-old liquor whole-
saler down in Nashville, likes to do. He started yoga to help him compete in the martial arts (and keep up with much younger guys). He's
not looking for a religious experience, and hasn't found one. "You
don't have to sit around and say 'Om' to do yoga," he says. "It doesn't
have to be all Eastern and mystical. To me, it's just the best workout,
bar none."

For us, yoga will be a tool for success, a way of reaching our goals,
and a competitive edge. Like they used to say about the U.S. Army—
now there's a comparison you never thought you'd hear—yoga helps

you be all you can be. One small component of this new Guy Yoga approach: I'm figuring you don't know Sanskrit. Am I right? So we won't be using all the exotic terminology that yoga folks sometimes love to throw around. What's the point of talking about two of the basic starting positions as "Tadasana" or "Shavasana," when you already know those two as Standing Up and Lying Down?

Before we hit the mats and get started, though, let me clear up one more thing. When you see yoga depicted on magazine covers or what-have-you, it's often some woman in a leotard looking really serene and contemplative. And it will relax your body and calm your mind.

Believe me, though, yoga can be hard. You're in for a demanding, athletically challenging workout here. Not bed-of-nails painful, just tough. Paul Hewitt, the men's basketball coach at Georgia Tech, started his players doing yoga a couple of seasons back. One thing he and his hoopsters found out, pronto: "This is not some passive, sit-around-and-contemplate kind of thing," the coach says. "It's very difficult, especially at first. It really stretches my guys to their limits."

But hey, hard is good, right? Real Men eat hard for breakfast. We know there's no free lunch; if you want to see results, you've gotta do the work.

Different is good, too. Before I started doing yoga a few years back, I'd been working out and playing sports my whole life, and my exercise routines had pretty much become ruts. (With the occasional knee or rotator cuff injury thrown in, just to keep things interesting.) So it's really been great to break out of the same-old same-old and put my body and concentration to new tests by doing yoga. And when I started to see myself getting better at it, I was proud: I really felt like I grew and that I accomplished something. You will too.

That reminds me—about that standing on-your-head thing I mentioned a while back: As I promised, you won't have to do that in this book, or the Shoulderstand or the Handstand. They're great, but kinda tricky; if you don't do them right, you can screw up your neck. So I'm going to skip them, and you can learn them with some hands-on instruction if you ever go to a yoga class.

If you do end up standing on your head one day, though, you know what? You just might like it. I learned to do it, and it's pretty cool. It's challenging and fun to look at the world a little differently—literally, since you're upside-down. And that holds true for yoga overall. Doing something new and getting a new perspective on your body and its capabilities are some of the best things a Real Man can get out of trying yoga.

All told, yoga offers physical and mental benefits that can make you a better athlete, a better worker, a better lover—in short, a healthier and happier dude. And yoga is something you can enjoy for the rest of your life. So what are you waiting for? Let's get started.

CHAPTER 1
Getting Started

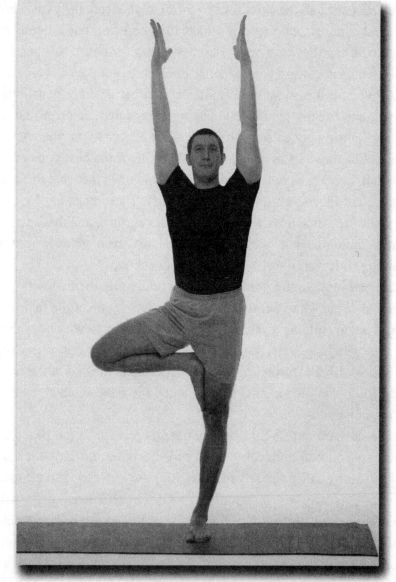

All you need to practice yoga is a non-slip surface and a little elbow room—
no special clothing or expensive equipment required. To nail this balancing
pose, you'll also need patience and a sense of fun.

A s you're about to see for yourself, yoga's a complex, sophisticated exercise system. Yet it's amazingly simple and easy to practice. You don't need any expensive equipment, and there's no gym or health club membership to pay for. Plus, you don't need all the extra time to travel to and from the gym: If you have 30 minutes total you can get a really good workout at home. For guys with families or who work crazy hours (or both), this can be a huge factor in getting your exercise done consistently.

All you need is some level floor space, either wood or nonslippery carpet, and I really recommend buying a yoga mat. You can find one in any sporting goods store these days for $20 or so, or you can buy 'em online at *yogajournal.com* (the Web site of the best yoga magazine out there) or at *huggermugger.com* (don't ask me what the name means, but they seem to make good stuff). These mats are "sticky," so you won't slide as you might on another surface, and that's important in holding your yoga positions. A mat also gives you some padding so it won't hurt your knees to kneel, etc.

Go barefoot; you're going to want to really grip the mat with your feet and dig in with your toes. This tactile feel is one of the first ways you'll begin building awareness of and connection to your body, head to toe. Clothing-wise, anything loose—T-shirts, your old baggy sweats—will do. During the relaxation period at the end of the workouts you'll cool down quickly, so it's good to have another dry layer or top at hand.

The only other thing you really need is privacy, some peace and quiet so you can concentrate. So tell the wife and kids that Dad needs some quality time by himself, kick out the dog, and close the door. TV is way too distracting, so no *SportsCenter;* sorry. After you've learned the positions and practiced for a while, you may find that music is a good accompaniment. For me, though, music interferes with the awareness and focus I'm trying to establish and makes it hard to follow my breathing. So I'd bag music, too, but see for yourself.

In a while, we'll learn the **Sun Salute,** the classic yoga warm-up we'll be using in our routines. But for now, before doing yoga just warm up and stretch for a few minutes however you usually do.

If you have any known health problems, including high blood pressure, heart disease or a spinal condition, check with your doctor before you begin a yoga program. If you have more run-of-the-mill sore spots like bad knees or an aching lower back—both common guy ailments—yoga may well help, but you should do the poses that involve your problems areas with caution. Ease your way in and out of them, especially when you're starting out.

Actually, that holds true for everyone. You're going to be moving your body in new ways, so take it easy on the old muscles and tendons; they have to last you a long time. Don't force your way into these stretches. You'll get "better"—that is, you will become more flexible and able to nail the poses more fully—over time. Don't try to make it all happen the first few times.

If at some point down the road you want to make your yoga workouts more strenuous or make certain poses more challenging, try staying in them longer rather than pushing or pulling yourself farther into them. You'll feel it, believe me, and you'll be a lot less likely to hurt yourself. *Pain is not gain. If doing any of these yoga moves hurts, stop or ease up.*

Take your time as you move through this book, learning all the poses one by one. Use the photos of our model, Glen de Vries, as your guide. Don't be surprised if some poses come really easily to you and others seem flat-out impossible. Everyone's different, and your weaker areas just tell you where the work is.

Remember to focus on your breathing, and coordinate breath and movements according to the instruction. In yoga, we breathe through the nose always, never with the mouth open. And if you don't, the Breath Police will come to your house and . . . just kidding! Obviously, you can breathe any way you want or feel you need to. It's a free country. But for reasons I'll explain in detail later, breathing is key to getting all yoga's great benefits. So for now, please just try to breathe the yoga way—when in Rome, and all that.

After you're comfortable with most of the moves, you can start following the first, shorter routine at the back of the book. But since that could take a while—and there's no rush, yoga isn't going anywhere—you can also work up to that by doing a mini-workout along the way. After you've learned the poses that promote upper body and lower body flexibility in chapters 2, 3 and 4, you can start doing those 10 poses together in roughly 10 minutes. You can do them just to practice but also to warm up; each time you pick up the book to learn more moves, do this Mini-Workout first. As you progress, add some strength and balance poses (your choice) from chapters 5 and 6. Then, after you learn the **Sun Salute** in chapter 9, make that the first thing you do each time you hit the mat.

Keep in mind, though, that the sequencing of yoga poses is important and adds considerable value. So when you get to the end of the book, make sure to switch over to the structured workouts—you'll get much better results.

Shoot for two sessions a week at first; then see if you can build to three. After a couple of months or so, you'll be ready to move up from the beginners or rookies workout to the more advanced veterans routine.

We'll start by looking at flexibility, something almost every guy I know could really use some help with. From stiff to Gumby, it all begins here. Enjoy.

CHAPTER 2

The Joy of Flex
& Why Yoga Flexes Best

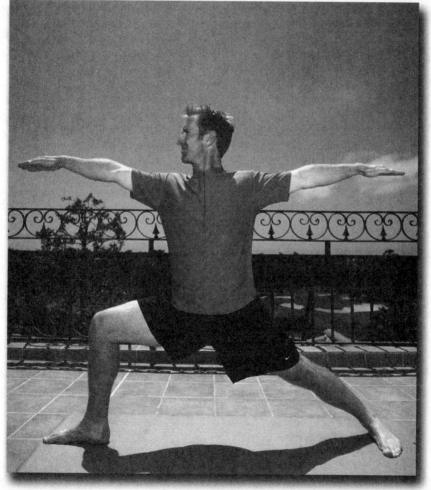

Joey Terrill/*Golf Digest*

PGA golfer David Duval, in the Warrior II stance. "I practice thirty minutes of yoga every day" he says, "for flexibility and strengthening the core muscles."

When most men think about flexibility . . . well, the truth is, we really don't think about it much at all. Why? For one thing, we equate flexibility with stretching—and stretching has got to be one of the most boring activities known to man. You lean against a wall, or bend, or pull some body part in a direction it doesn't really want to go, and basically wait for it to be over. Talk about tedious.

Plus, most guys simply aren't very flexible, especially compared to women. (You know we hate doing things we're not good at.) Unlike strength, flexibility doesn't really make you look good. Another reason guys aren't exactly enthralled with flexibility is that we don't really understand what good it does. Suppose you could bend over and touch your toes. How great would that really be? All these factors combine to make flexibility the major weakness in most men's fitness profiles.

But yoga will turn all that upside down. In this chapter and the next two, you'll see how stretching the yoga way completely blows away boredom. And no, being able to touch your toes isn't the ultimate goal. You'll begin to experience for yourself how improved flexibility will make you feel better, look better and perform better, right now and down the road when you're a Real Old Man.

First, while we're still young, some background on flexibility, including:

DEFINING THE F-WORD

Traditionally flexibility has meant the ability to lengthen the middle part or "belly" of a muscle to its ideal functional state. And yoga will help you with that, no question. Increasingly, though, sports scientists are realizing that developing more supple connective tissue—especially fascia—is also a vital flex factor. Tendons and ligaments are connective tissue, too; they support the whole muscle-bone-joint apparatus, holding it all in place. But they can't really be stretched or lengthened. When they are, that's an injury.

Fascia is where the give is. In an excellent *Yoga Journal* article on the science of flexibility, Fernando Pagés Ruiz explains that this connective tissue "makes up as much as 30 percent of a muscle's total mass, and . . . accounts for approximately 41 percent of a muscle's total resistance to movement." Yoga's deep, sustained stretches safely and effectively make fascia more limber—as well as the muscles themselves.

When muscles and connective tissue are lengthened and relaxed instead of bunched up (an inflexible muscle is a clenched, contracted muscle), that actually creates more room for blood to flow in and around them. Medical types call that "increased vascularity"; it just means more of the red stuff. More blood brings more oxygen, which muscles need to grow and heal. Increased circulation also helps to wash away lactic acid, a byproduct of muscle exertion—especially weightlifting—which can have a corrosive effect.

Plus, as your muscles finally relax into their full, proper length, your body—all 200-plus bones and 650-some muscles—gets aligned the way it's supposed to be. You'll be amazed, after doing yoga for a while, how much straighter you stand, naturally and effortlessly. "It's strange, but from my first yoga class eight years ago," says Craig Bromberg, a 40-something journalist in New York, "I actually felt like: 'I'm taller.'" It's a great feeling. And when the aches and pains that accompany inflexibility and misalignment disappear, you'll realize what a distraction and energy drain they were.

Flexibility also pays off big-time when it comes to sports. In fact, this is probably the biggest reason why athletes have been leading the charge to yoga. For one thing, the improved circulation we talked about helps jocks recover from getting banged up. Danny Poole teaches yoga to the University of Colorado football team and several players on the Denver Broncos (they call him "Yoga Danny"). "These football guys are sore for days after a game," says Poole. "They're so used to not feeling good, they think it's a fact of life. But then after we do an hour yoga session, they're like: 'Damn!' They can touch their toes again—and they just feel better. That's from opening the joints up and getting improved blood flow and circulation in the muscles, which heals injuries and bruises."

The reverse is also true: Being *inflexible* leads to injuries. Tight, contracted muscles pull on the bones they're attached to, restricting their movement and sometimes holding them out of place. Next thing you know, your humerus (arm bone to you) isn't sitting where it should be in its shoulder socket, to cite one common example. Over time, this creates an "impingement" and then an injury. Better flex nips this in the bud.

Listen to shooting guard **Wally Sczcerbiak** of the NBA's Minnesota Timberwolves. "Last year I really got into yoga before the season, just to get loose and stretch and to keep my body free from any lactic acids. It really helped me stay away from injuries, and I felt good the whole year. I think it's really helped my career." That was the 2001–2002 season he was talking about, in which he played all 82 games and made his first All-Star team.

Longer, more limber muscles perform better, with more spring and more strength. **Tanner Eriksen,** a right-handed pitcher in the Arizona Diamondbacks system who's been doing yoga since 2000, explains how it works in his sport. "In baseball," he says, "the longer the muscle, the more powerful. For pitching, you want to be long and loose, like a rubber band. That's what gives you good arm extension and when you're longer, you're getting more leverage." Tanner's 6'6", 240, so he's got some long levers working there. And his analysis is right on.

The reason is ROM. That stands for range of motion, and it's another way of saying "extension." What it means is that longer and more elastic muscles aren't just better in and of themselves, but that they also allow the joints—like a pitcher's shoulder—to rotate with greater mobility. Remember, those muscles are attached to bones, which insert into their sockets at the joints. When your shoulders, hips, elbows and knees can move more freely, the entire body moves better.

Makes sense (I hope), but you still may have a tough time seeing how being all loosey-goosey can actually make you stronger. Maybe more powerful is a better way to put it, and to explain that I'll have to take you back to Physics 101. Don't worry, it'll be quick. The key formula is: Force over distance equals power. So if either of those first two factors increases, so does the power output. When you get more movement (distance) in the joints, you generate more explosive force.

Dozens of top golfers on the PGA and LPGA tours now do yoga for flexibility and ROM (see the picture of **David Duval** that opens this chapter and chapter 11 on golf). They've learned that being able to rotate their shoulders and hips further—coiling and uncoiling their torsos more completely—lengthens the arc of their swings. That increased distance gives them more torque, more power. The payoff: longer drives.

Now that you're sold on flexibility, we can examine why yoga is hands-down the best way to get it. All the jocks you've been hearing from came to that conclusion—and these guys' bodies are worth millions of dollars. So they want to get the best performance from them for as long as they possibly can. To accomplish that, they want to use the best exercise techniques available. Don't you?

The Real Man

ANDY O'KEEFE

STOCKBROKER, 44, NEW YORK CITY

"I'm married, with seven kids. Been on Wall Street for 20 years. I'm the owner of a brokerage firm: 110 employees. I'm 6'4", 225 pounds. I've lifted weights for years and I run. I played lacrosse at college, and basketball, football in high school. So I love sports.

"A guy who sits next to me was dropping a lot of weight and telling me he was doing yoga. I was making fun of him. To tell the truth, he was getting quite a bit of ribbing from the rest of us. One night he grabbed me after work and said, 'Hey, you want to go with me, I got a class tonight.' I went. I came out of there—you know, I've been athletic my whole life—and I was never *so drained.* I felt so good. . . .

"I just thought yoga was: you sat there, meditated, stretched. That's all. I thought it was a weird Eastern thing. But that's not true at all. You know, I'm a believer.

"I feel stronger, more flexible. And it's helped me with golf. I still lift weights twice a week, but with yoga, I feel much looser. Mentally, it kind of clears your head. You can't think about anything but what you're doing while you're in there. It's a good escape for me.

"Now about five or six of us guys from the office go. I wish I had more time; if I did, I would do yoga five times a week."

WHY YOGA FLEXES BEST

So that you can really understand—and better yet, *feel*—how yoga is light years ahead of old-school stretching, we're going to do a one-on-one comparison right now, including your first yoga position. So get ready to rumble!

You see, the way that most of us have been taught to stretch isolates specific muscles in what exercise physiologists call "static" or passive stretching. But yoga moves don't just isolate one muscle for stretching—they're much more complex and demand more from your body and your mind.

Holding a yoga stance gently lengthens an entire group of interdependent muscles and at the same time calls in an opposing set of muscles to support the first bunch by contracting. (For those of you keeping score at home, the first bunch are known as the "agonists" and the corresponding group are the "antagonists.") To maintain yoga positions, you'll also need to call on the body's legions of (mostly smaller) stabilizer muscles. Not to get all yoga-jargony on you, but they're "integrated" movements.

To demonstrate the difference, we'll do one of each kind of stretch right now. Let's say you're getting ready to pump some iron, and you want to stretch out your chest first. Here's how you'd do it the traditional way—and then the yoga way.

Old School

Stand in an open doorway. Feet are parallel, or one in front of the other; doesn't matter. Raise both arms to shoulder height, elbows bent, and catch the door frame on both sides with your forearms and elbows. Now lean your head and torso forward through the doorway, pushing your chest out to create a stretch across your pecs. Hold that for 30 seconds (45 seconds if you're over 40).

What happened? Well, hopefully, your pecs got a little looser, and that's good. But the opposing muscles, on your back, might as well have been asleep. And the doorway was holding you up, so you didn't have to balance yourself or concentrate much to maintain your position—in fact, you might as well have been asleep, period.

Time to wake up and try a chest stretch the yoga way.

New School

This chest opener is one of the great yoga postures, known as the **Cobra.** *You can see from the accompanying photo where it gets the name—in it you look kinda like one of those hooded snakes with its head up, ready to strike.*

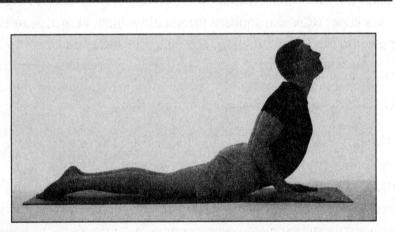

◆ Lie face down on the mat with your legs stretched back, tops of the feet on the floor. Feet and inner thighs are close together.

◆ Put your palms on the floor to the sides of your shoulders, and spread the fingers wide. You're in a pre-pushup position. Keep the hand muscles engaged and active and the elbows tucked in close to your body.

◆ Inhale as you begin to lift your chest off the floor and arch your torso backward, straightening the arms roughly halfway to three quarters (don't lock the elbows out). Try to use the spine, plus the back and chest muscles to do the lifting more than the arms. Don't lift the hips off the floor, just the upper body. You want to feel a good stretch across the front of your chest.

◆ As you come up, tighten the muscles in your butt a little to support your lower back. Press your legs and the tops of the feet down into the floor to get more oomph behind your torso's upward thrust. Look up at the ceiling, or if that's uncomfortable, straight ahead.

◆ Don't overdo the backbend. Come up only as far as is comfortable with reasonable effort. To find the right height for you and avoid straining your back, take your hands off the floor for a moment and see where you can comfortably hold without them. Then put the hands back down. Six inches off the ground is okay. And try to arch your upper back and squeeze the shoulder blades together to help form the bend; don't just scrunch into your lower back.

◆ Hold the pose for 5 slow breaths (5 inhales and 5 exhales).

◆ On an exhale, release back down to the floor.

(Note: If this pose bothers your lower back, either don't come up as far and/or place your hands farther forward on the floor. If it still hurts, skip it. *Yoga shouldn't hurt.*)

Feels pretty active, right? Not "static" at all. That's because you were not only stretching the pecs, opening the chest nicely, as you did in the doorway, but also working the back muscles, retracting the shoulder girdle and engaging the lats, the lower traps and the rhomboids. The forearms and the triceps got a wake-up call and the legs muscles were energized, too. Plus, you were flexing the entire spine in a backbend, a very powerful yoga motion.

As you probably noticed, it's a challenge. Stretching the yoga way, there's no doorway, no wall or park bench to help you. *You* have to do all the work, and there's a lot more of it.

Boredom? Forget about it. You had to really bear down and concentrate, right? When you get better at these more difficult yoga moves—and you will, because they are just the right mix of difficult and doable—it will feel great because you'll have really accomplished something. I ask you: Did you ever feel that way about stretching?

Let's move on and learn some more poses that promote flexibility in the upper body. Odds are they'll really help you; lots of guys are pretty immobile upstairs from working out with weights (trying to look like Real Men). And congratulations, by the way: By doing that one **Cobra** pose, you're now officially a yogi.

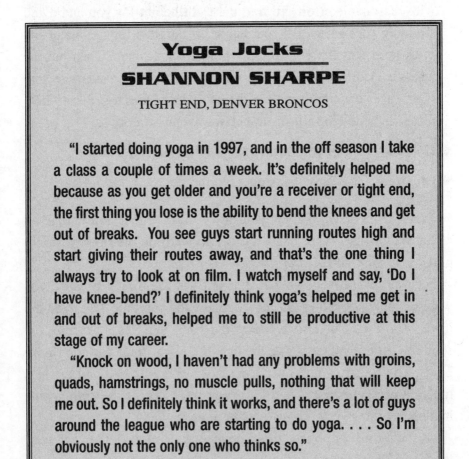

Yoga Jocks
SHANNON SHARPE
TIGHT END, DENVER BRONCOS

"I started doing yoga in 1997, and in the off season I take a class a couple of times a week. It's definitely helped me because as you get older and you're a receiver or tight end, the first thing you lose is the ability to bend the knees and get out of breaks. You see guys start running routes high and start giving their routes away, and that's the one thing I always try to look at on film. I watch myself and say, 'Do I have knee-bend?' I definitely think yoga's helped me get in and out of breaks, helped me to still be productive at this stage of my career.

"Knock on wood, I haven't had any problems with groins, quads, hamstrings, no muscle pulls, nothing that will keep me out. So I definitely think it works, and there's a lot of guys around the league who are starting to do yoga. . . . So I'm obviously not the only one who thinks so."

CHAPTER 3
Flexing the Upper Body & the Spine

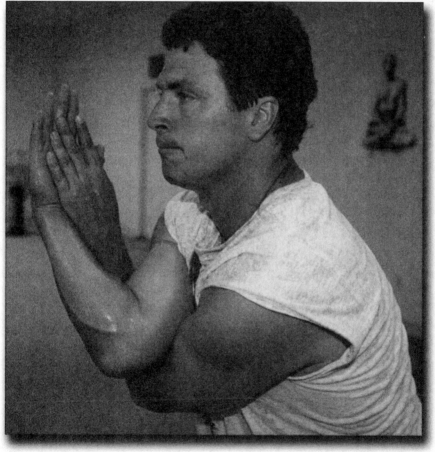

Bill Frakes/*Sports Illustrated*

All-time great quarterback Dan Marino took up yoga after an Achilles injury. The position he's working here, the Eagle, is a great upper-body stretch.

Eddie George is one strong man. A Heisman Trophy winner at Ohio State, he's a 6'3", 235-pound running back for the NFL's Tennessee Titans. Even in that league of bulging behemoths, he's known for the intensity of his training and his powerful body. But Eddie's got a sensitive, vulnerable side.

No, we're not talking about his emotions or his psyche. This vulnerability is to injury. Like all running backs, George gets tackled at the end of most every play and gets pinned under a stack of linemen, defenders and other pilers-on that can easily weigh more than one thousand pounds. Ouch. That's like having six or seven sofas stacked on top of you, only these crazed couches would just as soon hurt you as not. "It can get pretty vicious in there," Eddie says with a laugh.

Being at the bottom of the pileup is even more dangerous, he explains, because "I often land in twisted, awkward positions. And just a little tweak can mean an injury. I wanted to try to beat those odds and by doing so get a competitive edge."

So five years ago George sought out Nashville yoga teacher Hilary Lindsay and began working with her two or three times a week. He's kept up these private sessions ever since. Remember, five years ago yoga was nowhere near as popular in this country, especially among men. It was still a pretty out-there thing to do. But George had the foresight to cut through the hype and try it for himself. "When I first tried it, it was extremely tough, very hard, just getting in the poses," he remembers. "But now I really enjoy doing it. I just knew it would increase flexibility and decrease the chances of getting hurt."

Sure looks that way. George has been a workhorse, never missing a start in seven seasons. During that time he gained more yards running than any other back in the league and was named to the Pro Bowl four straight times. "Yoga's definitely helped my durability," he says. "Now if I'm put in an awkward position on the field, my muscles have already experienced something like that stretch before, in yoga. If I was tight, I might get a pull or a bone might break."

FLEX TEST: The Upper Body

To get a sense of how flexible—or how stiff—you are in the upper body, take this assessment used by Paul Frediani, a New York trainer who is also the author of four books on flexibility (*Golf Flex, Ski Flex, Surf Flex* and *Sex Flex*).

- Raise your right arm, then bend your elbow and reach down behind your back and try to touch the top of your left shoulder blade.
- Then take your left arm, extended downward, bend it at the elbow and reach upward behind your back to touch the bottom of the right shoulder blade.
- And vice-versa.

If you can do both, on both sides, you're doing good. If not, you see where you have room for improvement.

If you have really good flexibility, you'll be able to do the following. This is actually a yoga move called, for some unfathomable reason, **Cow Face**:

- Extend your right arm up, then bend it at the elbow, dropping your hand down the center of your upper back to the area between the shoulder blades (or as far as you can reach).
- Reach your left arm behind your back, elbow at waist level, and come up from below to meet the other hand— just clasping fingers, not a handshake—in the middle of your back. Then try the reverse. You may only be able to do this one way, but don't worry. If you can even get your fingers to touch, you're up there in the higher flexibility percentiles. To work on this, hold a towel between your hands and gently pull them together.

George's upper body is vulnerable because of the way running backs play. "Your upper body is basically a battering ram," Eddie says. Crashing into defenders—and vice versa—means absorbing tremendous hits to the shoulders, head and neck. Add in the fact that his torso was hyper-developed from weightlifting, and you can see why having mobility in his shoulder joints and being able to rotate his torso are major priorities. To address that, Lindsay taught him the **Cobra** and other poses we're going to learn here. One unexpected side effect of their training together: "He got flexible, but I got really strong," laughs Hilary. "I had to hold up this 240-pound man in balancing poses. You should see my arms!"

Seeing is believing. After the Titans saw the benefits of yoga in Eddie George, they called in Lindsay before the 2002 season to work with the entire team.

THE REAL MAN

Okay, you're no Eddie George. No offense, but odds are you're not in his class as a physical specimen. And you probably don't face the same kinds of occupational hazards. But we weekend warriors can gain as much flexibility from yoga as the pros—or even more, since they're often in fantastic shape to begin with. Like this next Real Man did.

Jerry Grossman used to ache for days after playing basketball. "I had a lot of pain in my shoulders, up in the rotator cuff area, from reaching really high or back over my head for a rebound," says the 43-year-old New Yorker. He and some of the other guys in his regular game would pop Advil *before and after* hitting the hoops.

The problem was "my shoulders and chest were naturally tight, and then I made it more so, probably, by lifting weights," Grossman says. After pumping iron at the gym one day four years ago, Grossman wandered into a yoga class. "It drew me in immediately," he says. For one thing, he's single, and "there are a lot more women than men in these classes, and they look good." But let's get back to flexibility.

Grossman began taking classes three times a week. "It took a lot of hard work, but my shoulders and chest have really opened up," Jerry says. His ROM has improved tremendously: "I can reach places on my back that I could never touch before." And that shows up on the court. Grossman says his newfound reach "definitely helps me in rebounding and in shot-blocking." And the pain is gone—no more Advil. "I used to have to baby myself for a couple of days after I worked out hard, but now I don't give it a moment's thought. I can really bounce right back."

So now he's telling all his hoops buddies about yoga, right? Well, not exactly. Seems Grossman's one of those guys who likes to keep yoga a secret—that's *his* competitive edge. "Every once in a while I'll tell someone at the game how to stretch better," he says. "But mostly I just sort of smile to myself. . . ."

Sorry, Jerry. And you, too, Eddie George. We're about to give away the secrets of your success. Here are three more yoga poses that will limber up your upper half. I think you're really going to enjoy getting more flexible, and you'll feel looser and more relaxed once you do. But if by any chance you don't like these exercises, you can have all your old stiffness back, no questions asked.

CAT STRETCH

A nice easy one to get started with, and yet an effective ice-breaker: A few rounds of this will give you a good idea of where you're tight in the upper chest, back and spine, and will gently begin melting 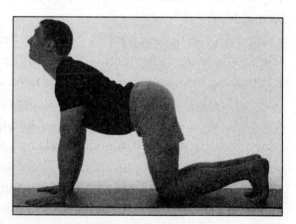 that tightness away. This two-part stretch also engages and tones the

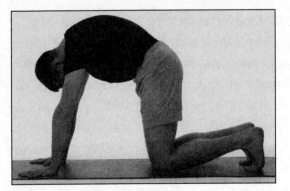

back muscles around the shoulder blades.

◆ Get down on the mat on all fours, arms straight. (You pretty much never want to lock your elbows or knees in yoga.) Head is in a neutral position; you're looking at the ground.

◆ Breathe in slowly, and keeping your hands and knees in the same places, tilt your upper chest upward and sink your lower back downward at the same time, creating a mild U-shape curve in the spine. Look up, raising your head. You'll note that your butt is now sticking way out and up—good thing no one's looking. Get a good stretch here, but don't force anything.

◆ Now reverse the stretch. Exhale slowly as you tuck your head down (now you're looking back at your feet), lengthening the neck and rounding your shoulders and back upward (like a cat stretching). Now the spinal curve is the other way, more of a dome-like shape.

◆ Repeat 4 more times, very slowly. Then relax.

THE HALF EAGLE

Sounds a little odd? Okay, you got me—I made this one up. But bear with me. This wraparound move is half of a great balancing pose we'll learn later in the book. But I've found that, minus the balancing and lower body component, it's a terrific stretch for the back and shoulders. So let's just do this bird halfway now and do the full **Eagle** down the road. For extra inspiration, check out the picture of football great **Dan Marino** in the **Eagle** that opens this chapter.

◆ Standing up, raise both arms in front of you, elbows bent, so your upper and lower arms form 90-degree angles. The undersides of your upper arms are parallel with the floor.

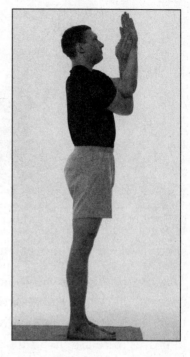

◆ Place the left elbow inside the bend of the right one. Snake the right forearm around and behind the left forearm so they are intertwined, "braided" together. Press your right fingers against your left palm, both hands pointing straight up.

◆ Now inhale and lift your elbows up together, as close to shoulder height as possible. As you do so, lift the chin and chest as close to vertical as possible. The tendency here is to bring the head down and hunch forward, but you want to stand up as straight as possible. Feel the stretch this puts into your back muscles.

◆ Hold for 30 seconds, breathing slowly and fully.

◆ Unwrap the arms, then shake them out. Then reverse the starting positions of the arms and repeat.

Those first two poses weren't so traumatic, right? Good, because things are gonna get more intense.

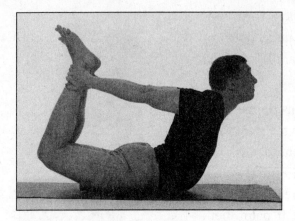

THE BOW

Think archery here. Your arms will play the part of the bowstrings, and drawing them tighter will supply the tension that bends the bowstaff: your trunk. This move is a great compensator for all the forward bending we do at work (over the computer) and at play (any sport in which your movement and momentum are mostly forward).

The **Bow** really opens up your front, especially the shoulders and upper chest, while strengthening the "antagonists" in the upper and lower back (you'll feel a strong stretch in the quads also). And it improves the elasticity of the spine. Just give this a few gentle tries— no yanking!—you'll soon be amazed at how good it feels to flex "the wrong way" and how bendy you've suddenly become. You're gonna be a regular Gumby!

◆ Lie face down on the mat, arms and legs extended.

◆ Bend the legs at the knees. Keep your lower abdomen flat on the mat.

◆ Reach the arms back and grab your ankles with both hands, palms facing in. Your forehead is still on the mat.

◆ Inhale and lift your legs, chest and head off the mat. Your head is now erect, face forward. Press your feet and lower legs away from your core, pulling against the arms. This tension in both directions (your arms are drawing your legs forward at the same time) will help raise your chest and open the shoulders—you're bending the **Bow**. You can accentuate the upper body stretch by drawing your shoulder blades together in the center of your back. The chest muscles are now stretched pretty tight, so make sure to breathe fully.

◆ Hold for 5 full breaths.

◆ Exhale, release your ankles, and slowly lower your legs and chest.

◆ Rest and repeat twice, trying to raise a little bit more of your body off the floor each time. But don't go too hard, and if you feel any pain in your lower back, quit. Remember, Real Men don't force it.

Next we're going to explore a component of upper-body flexibility unique to yoga, one that most exercise methods ignore: bending the very core of the torso, the spine.

FLEXING THE SPINE

It's an amazing design: a vertical stack of bite-size vertebrae surrounded by muscles and those gelatinous sacs, the discs. This flexible, segmented rod moves every which way, allowing you to bend forward, backward, left, right and rotate in all those directions. To understand what a truly flexible spine allows, picture those young female gymnasts who can bend their little bodies almost beyond belief. The reason is, at that age, their spines are basically Jell-O. And as their spines stiffen at about age 16 or so, they can no longer compete at the highest level.

This happens to us guys, too, of course. With age, inactivity and/or injury, we lose spinal flexibility. Now picture an old man. You know how lots of old guys have that hunched-over, almost humpbacked way they stand, with their heads sunken down into their chests? That's calcification, when the discs and vertebrae compress, and the exaggerated forward curve in the upper back is called "kyphosis." It's not a good look, is it? Well, that's the look of a man who's been inflexible in his upper body for a long, long time. Like, say, you, if you don't get your act together. As Joseph Pilates—inventor of another exercise regimen men are leery of—said, "You are as young as your spinal column."

The good news is: Yoga is Viagra for the spine. In yoga classes they often tell you to try to roll up or down on your back "vertebra by vertebra," and after a while, you actually feel that you can do it, that you can approximate that kind of segment-by-segment elasticity.

When your spine is flexible, you have greater ROM in all the directions the spine moves. And keeping the spine strong through exercise will also help you ward off osteoporosis (yes, men have it too). Starting now, both of these qualities will serve you long and well in your everyday activities and of course, in sports, especially golf.

We've already been flexing the spine in some of the poses we've learned: The **Bow** has you bending backward and **Cobra** is obviously a backbend. Here are a couple spinal twists to really give that apparatus a tune-up.

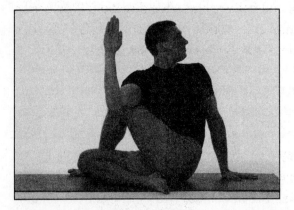

SEATED TWIST

◆ Sit on the floor or mat cross-legged. If your knees are way up in the air, don't worry—we'll deal with that later, when we work on lower-body flexibility.

◆ Pick the left foot up off the floor and step it over the right leg, placing it sole-down just outside the right thigh. The left knee is now pointing straight up.

◆ Take a big inhale and lift and straighten the torso, lifting the head straight up as well. "Grow the spine!" as some yoga folks put it.

◆ Exhale and twist the trunk to the left. Have the trunk initiate the action, not the head and neck.

◆ Now lift the right arm, bent at the elbow, then reach it over and place the back of the elbow on the outside of the left knee. This is your control lever with which you can adjust the extent of the twist. The right hand is open, fingers pointing straight up at the ceiling.

◆ Breathe! Take deep inhales, and as you do, try to straighten up more or make yourself more erect from the hips up. On the exhales, try to twist around just a little bit more to the left, pushing off the knee with the back of the elbow.

◆ Continue for 6 to 8 breaths, then release.

◆ Reverse the positions of the feet and the rotation of the twist.

SUPER-CHARGE IT!

To twist the torso farther around, imagine as you begin to rotate, that you are moving the navel and belly in the same direction. Whether or not those parts actually move, it works. Again, don't lead with your head and neck to twist more deeply; you might strain your neck.

THE KNEELING TWIST

Here's a variation they teach at the Dharma Yoga Center in New York City. The kneeling stance gives you more stability and torque to get a good twist, and it brings a little bit of a balance challenge with it to keep you alert.

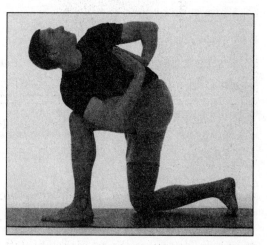

◆ Sit up on the mat, resting on both knees with your lower legs out behind you.

◆ Swing the left leg out in front of you, bend at the knee and rest the left foot about 8 inches farther out than the right knee.

◆ Inhale deeply and shoot the right arm straight up overhead, more or less in line with that ear.

◆ Now exhale slowly and bend forward at the waist, reaching across with your right arm, bending it at the elbow and catching that right elbow on the outside of your left knee. Just get a feel for that, then:

◆ Drop down farther and twist your trunk back and to the left, so you're now facing left. Slide the inside of the right arm as far down the left leg as it will go—ideally, you will end up with your right armpit draped over the left knee and you'll be able to hold yourself stable there with that bind, knee pinned between the chest and back of the right arm. Your head will come forward and down as you do this. (Better look at the picture.)

◆ Now bring your left arm forward to meet the right, pressing the palms strongly together. Both forearms should now form a straight line, and you can use them as a unit, swinging them up and to the left more to deepen the twist.

◆ When you've turned as far as you can, turn your head and try to look back and up at the ceiling. If it bothers your neck, drop this part.

◆ Hold yourself in the twist and breathe deeply. If you feel yourself keeling over to one side, move the back leg that's on the ground as needed to create a more stable platform.

◆ After 5 full breaths, inhale and untwist.

◆ Repeat on other side.

Learning moves like these, it's really striking how neatly—wonderfully—all your different parts can fit and function together. You gotta give those old Indian guys credit: They thought up so many ingenious ways to use and improve the human body. Give the body credit, too, for being able to do so many incredible things. Finally, give yourself some credit: When you first see these twists—and the Bow—being done, they can look way too difficult and completely out-of-reach. But if you just give them some repeated, gentle tries (no yanking!) you'll soon be surprised at how flexible and competent you've become. The human body is amazing—and you've got a good one!

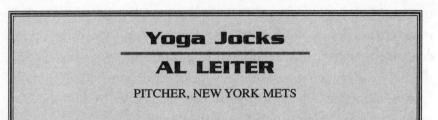

Yoga Jocks

AL LEITER

PITCHER, NEW YORK METS

"I tried yoga in 1990 after my second arm operation, thinking that conventional workouts weren't working. It was a great workout, and I realized after that most athletes aren't very flexible. You get in the weight room and do your bench press, your curls, your back and lats—but you don't stretch enough.

"I do Bikram Yoga and it's an intense hour-and-a-half routine of 26 poses—in a room that's 100 degrees. You sweat and your heart rate is pounding; it's one of the hardest workouts I've ever done in my life.

"It helps my whole body. My joints feel better, my knees. It helps in my range of motion and my flexibility is greater.

"I do very little hypnotic and meditation stuff. That might get a little too far left for me. There are some things I take from the breathing exercises, because a consistent breathing pattern brings oxygen to the muscles and therefore puts your body in optimum position to succeed. And I do think that yoga's also a lot of mind therapy, trying to fight through fatigue to hold the poses.

"During the winter I do it twice a week. And then during the season I do one workout between every start. It is absolutely the best, no bullshit. If there is anybody out there who's thinking 'Maybe I'll try it,' absolutely, try it. It is awesome."

CHAPTER 4
Flexing the Lower Body

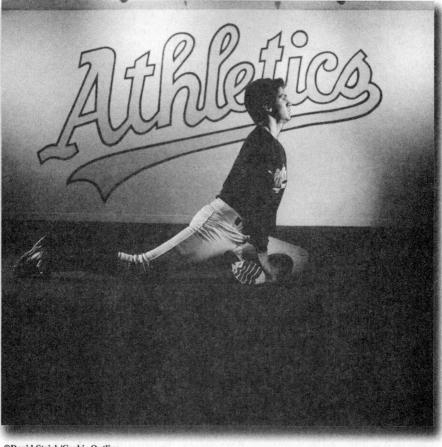

©David Strick/Corbis Outline

Barry Zito, one of baseball's premier pitchers, beginning the Pigeon, a powerful hip opener. Zito uses yoga and meditation to help him prepare for every game.

FLEXIBILITY: THE LOWER BODY

We guys really have it bad here. If you've ever watched women stretch, you've probably noticed how open and loose they are in their lower halves. They can sit cross-legged and their knees somehow settle down to rest on the floor. Meanwhile, if you can even touch your manly toes, odds are you've been doing yoga. More often than not, our hips, groins and hamstrings are criminally tight.

Dr. Craig Aaron, a yoga instructor and chiropractor who works with the Georgia Tech men's basketball team, jokes that "When the guys first sat on the floor cross-legged for me, their knees were shooting up toward their ears." And those guys are 18-year-old athletes; you'd think they'd be way more flexible than you and me. What gives?

Partly it's differences in anatomy, but a lot of it has to do with how we use our lower muscles and joints. All that driving around in the car and sitting on our butts in the office chair are basically invitations for our leg muscles to shorten and tighten. But it's not just inactivity to blame—our activities tighten us up, too. Almost every form of exercise or sport we play involves running (or skating), which puts pressure on the feet, ankles, knees and hips. Even golf requires repeated hip rotation, stressing those joints and muscles. As for those Georgia Tech hoopsters, Aaron explains that: "There's a lot of pounding of the hips in basketball, especially from jumping so high and then landing hard. So we need do a lot of hip openers with them."

All this repeated stress can lead to pain, stiffness and injuries. For the lower body to compensate, recover and function optimally, it takes better flexibility than most guys have. The good news is: You can do it. Yoga will loosen up and invigorate everything from your hamstrings down to your toes. Just listen to this success story:

After Ken Canfield, a trial lawyer based in Atlanta, had been taking Ashtanga yoga classes for about a year, the health club where he does his other workouts offered all its clients a flexibility test. Like our Flex Test (see box), it measured how far each person could reach forward toward their toes in a seated position. "The best score among all the customers was a 37," Canfield reports, his voice starting to rise as if even he can't believe what happened. "Then all the trainers took the test and the best score among all of them was a 39." And his score, pray tell? "I got a 43," he laughs. "And here's the thing: I'm 50 years old. I'm 15 or 20 years older than the rest of them!"

When you talk to pro athletes who've gotten into yoga, lower-body flexibility is often Job One. Here's **Mike Lieberthal,** a two-time All-Star for the Philadelphia Phillies, who's been doing yoga two to three times a week for many years:

"I'm a catcher, and flexibility is one thing we really need. We do a lot of ups and downs and squatting. That wears on you. We especially need flexibility in the groin, because after you squat you have to be able to move really quick to the right or left, depending on if a pitch is on the inside or the outside corner. It's like a goalie in hockey, moving to stop a shot. And after I'd been doing yoga, I found it was a lot easier to get up and down on my legs—the movements come more easily."

Speaking of hockey goalies, **Sean Burke** of the Phoenix Coyotes started doing yoga about four years ago for just the reasons that Lieberthal describes. You've seen how goalies splay their lower legs outward as they drop down to their knees on the ice to block shots with those big pads. Well, that move, called the butterfly, "takes a lot of energy and effort," Burke says, "and after a while, it affects your hips, your back, your hamstrings, your groin. So I tried the yoga, and I haven't had many problems in those areas at all since."

FLEX TEST: The Lower Body

Here's a quick, easy way to see how loose or tight you are in the lower back and hamstrings, adapted from material from the American College of Sports Medicine.

- Warm up and stretch lightly before you begin. Then sit on the floor with your legs outstretched in front of you.
- Grab a yardstick and put it on the floor between your legs with the low markings (0 inches) closer to you, and your heels at the 15-inch mark. Your feet should be about 10 inches apart.
- Place one hand over the other with one middle finger on top of its twin.
- Slowly stretch forward without jerking or bouncing, and slide your fingertips along the yardstick as far as possible. Do this three times and remember the highest number you reach. That's your score.

Here's how you rate among men (yup, women do better), based on your age:

Age	Score
20–29	19 or over = high; 13–18 = average
30–39	18 or over = high; 12–17 = average
40–49	17 or over = high; 11–16 = average
50–59	16 or over = high; 10–15 = average

"Plus, I think I'm a much better goaltender because of it," Burke says. I have better flexibility now than I ever have had in my life, and I've got a wider butterfly position now. When I drop down and stretch both legs out to stop a shot, I cover more net. Honestly, we've measured it and I think my butterfly is eight inches wider than it used to be. And I'm getting down on the ice more quickly. No question, you're going to make more saves like that."

It's paid off for Burke, on the ice and off. Over the last three seasons he's completely revived his career; in the 2001–2002 season he made his third All-Star team. His improved performance earned him a fat multiyear contract extension, at age 35. "Yoga's definitely a reason why things have gone so well for me," Burke says, "I truly believe that yoga has been a huge part of my success." (To hear more of his take on yoga, see the Yoga Jocks sidebar in this chapter.)

It'll pay off for you too. The way I look at it, since this is the biggest problem area for so many guys, it's also the area in which you can make the greatest gains—this is where yoga will help you the most. And when your legs, hips and lower back (there'll be more on this in the chapter on back pain) finally loosen up, you are going to love the way it feels. As far as that "yoga glow" goes, this is the mother lode.

We'll start with the hammies, which, if you're an active guy at all, are probably winched pretty tight. So we'll go slowly. You may already be familiar with this first simple stretch from your jock days. We'll use a strap to ease our way into it. A ratty towel or old belt will do; even surgical tubing. If you want to go a little more upscale, there is such a thing as a stretching strap, usually cotton or canvas.

Listen up: This may seem like a one-legged pose all the way. But here and with all the similar moves, it's very important that you put the "off leg" to work, keeping it strong by engaging the muscles, charging them with effort and energy. This technique will actually make the poses a lot easier and more effective. It's something that our technical consultant, Michael Lechonczak, always emphasizes in his classes: "Muscle energy!" Put more in and you'll get more out.

Besides the hamstrings, this exercise will gently loosen your groin, hip and calf muscles. In Yoga-ese, it's **Reclining Big Toe Pose,** but we'll just call it:

HAMSTRING STRETCH

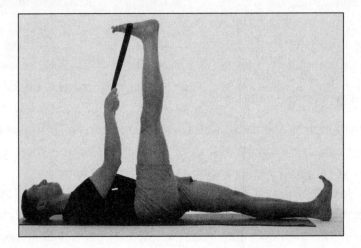

◆ Lying on your back with your legs extended, draw your right leg up toward your chest, knee bent, and loop the strap around the arch or the ball of your right foot. (I find using the ball gives me a little better torque when I'm pulling the leg back; see what works best for you.) Hold onto the ends of the strap with one hand or two, it doesn't matter.

◆ On an inhale, straighten the right leg, then try to raise it straight up, at a right angle to your body. Really flexible folks (mostly women) will be able to pull the leg back toward their heads and bring the ankle to the face. Most likely that's not you at this stage of the game; just let the leg stop where it needs to.

◆ Push up with the heel, flexing the foot back, then extend the foot forward, pointing the toes a few times for a preliminary stretch. End with the foot relaxed and basically flat.

◆ Check in on the other leg, the one that's lying flat on the ground. The first thing to check is that it still is lying flat; don't let it come up as you raise the other leg. But it shouldn't be just lying there. Make sure it's alive with muscle energy.

◆ Breathe slowly and deeply through your nose. Relax the tension on the strap a little on the inhales; then, on the exhales, try to pull it a little tighter, moving the leg back more toward your chest and head. You should feel this stretch in your hamstrings. Don't move your trunk toward the leg; make sure your shoulders, upper back and head all stay flat on the floor. Do this for 10 breaths.

◆ Exhale, release the strap and lower the leg.

◆ Repeat on the other side.

Real Men Don't: Pull too hard, too soon. We're shooting for incremental progress here, over the course of many workouts. Trying to yank the leg way back like a showgirl in Session One is not advised.

DOWNWARD DOG

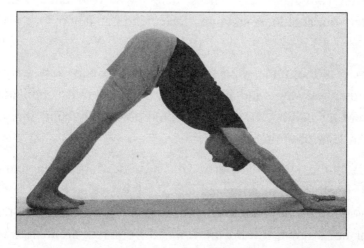

This is one of the best and most enjoyable overall stretches in yoga. It's terrific for the upper body, but for me—and, I suspect, a lot of other guys with lower body "issues"—the greatest benefit is the gentle stretch you get along the entire back of your lower half, from the top of your butt down to the arches of your feet. And, in the complex way yoga works, you're also strengthening the muscles on the front of your legs and working the arms while you're at it.

The **Downward Dog** is both a loosener and a rejuvenator—it feels great, right off the bat. Maybe that's why you see dogs, this pose's namesakes, putting the old snout down and the back end up. (If you don't have a dog you can just refer to the human in the picture.) Hey, if it's good enough for Bowser . . .

Reminder: As these positions get tougher and the muscles begin to really feel stressed, we tend to hold our breath. But that's actually when you need to keep breathing the most, slowly and deeply.

◆ Get on your hands and knees, then move your hands out from under your shoulders so your arms extend out at about a 45-degree angle.

◆ Tuck your toes under your feet and, as you exhale, start straightening out your legs and lifting your butt and midsection upward toward the ceiling. Your knees should be slightly bent, and you're up on your toes.

◆ Then on the next exhale, drop your head down between your arms and straighten your arms and legs (both extended but not locked), so you're pushing back onto your feet and your weight is pressing your heels down toward the floor. If your feet aren't flat on the floor, don't worry. That remaining distance is just the flexibility you are about to gain. You should feel the stretch in your hammies, calves and Achilles. Maintain here for 5 full breaths, in and out.

◆ Now exhale and bow your upper half down closer to the floor, dropping the head and torso down between the arms till you feel the stretch in your upper torso and front shoulders. Now you're working everything at once. Take 5 more slow breaths.

◆ Return your focus to the backs of the legs. To stretch them out a little more, inhale and come back up on your toes, then while exhaling, push your heels back down toward the floor. Repeat 3 times.

◆ Okay, you're a Done Dog. Take a rest, boy.

Real Men Don't: Let all the torso's weight fall on the wrists; they can get strained. To avoid that, spread out the fingers wide, broadening the palms, and try to take the weight on the fleshy part of your palms. Stretching the hands out like this will also activate the forearms and biceps; you want them awake and involved, too.

CRESCENT MOON

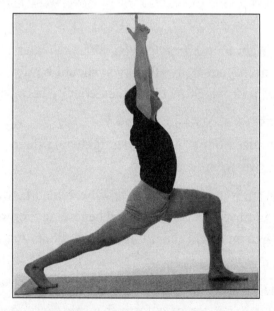

You'll definitely feel this stretch in your groin, but it also does great work on the hip flexors and the psoas. The what? The psoas (pronounced so-az) is a deep interior muscle that runs from the inside of your thigh bone, underneath the hip flexors, all the way to the lower back where it connects to the lumbar spine. It's a very important stabilizer that promotes mobility in the hips. In fact, Colorado yoga teacher Katherine Roberts, calls the psoas "the key to golf." (To see how she backs up that statement, check out chapter 12.)

Though we're focusing here on lower-body flexing, **Crescent Moon** is also a nice backbend. As you can see in the picture, the goal is to sink down, bend back and swoop the arms overhead so the line arching from your back foot upward to the hands creates a crescent-moon-shaped curve.

Note: You'll see in the accompanying photo that Glen, our yoga model, likes to do this pose with his knee up, off the ground. You can try that in a while, but for the most part I recommend keeping the knee down on the mat, as per the instructions below.

◆ Start kneeling on the mat with your torso erect, arms down at your sides.

◆ Place your right foot in front of you, about two and a half or three feet away from your body. The knee should be directly over the right ankle. Your weight is distributed equally between your front and back legs.

◆ Inhale and raise both arms high, straightening them and clasping your hands over your head.

◆ Exhale and shift your lower torso downward and forward, shifting the weight out over the front foot and beginning the stretch in your left groin area and right inner thigh. Keep the left/back leg where it is.

◆ As you sink forward into the stretch, draw the arms farther back, arching your upper torso to form that crescent-moon curve and intensify the stretch in the groin area. As you move, turn your face upward and look at your clasped hands, dropping the head back to do so. Don't go nuts here; moving the hands back just six inches or so will do it.

◆ Take five complete, slow breaths. Then on the next inhale, shift your weight back to the left leg and relax the stretch, lowering the arms.

◆ Now bring the left leg out front and do the other side.

SUPER-CHARGE IT!

As you get looser in this area, you can deepen the stretch by taking the back knee off the ground and turning your stance into a lunge (see photo). This way you're stretching the quadriceps in the back leg as well as the hips and groin area, plus you have to balance your body to keep it from falling to either side, so the pose gets more challenging. Don't forget to look up at the hands—and breathe!

The Pigeon can be a tough one for us Tight Guys. It's a tremendously powerful hip opener and a great stretch for the butt muscles, or glutes—among the biggest and strongest in the body. Once you're able to get into it deeply, it will also stretch the piriformus muscle, a deep internal rotator in the butt which, if gets clenched, can contribute to sciatica.

Because it's such a nuclear-powered move, it's one of the favorites of pro athletes, whose big muscles get extra tight and who need to counter the constant pounding on their lower bodies. Eddie George of the Titans says, "Pigeon's my thing. It opens up the hips, and I really need mobility there. When I first tried it, it was extremely tough; now I can get all the way down there. It allows me to move better and feel better doing it."

Alan Jaeger has run a six-week off-season yoga camp for baseball players in California since 1993. Mike Lieberthal of the Phillies and

Cy Young award-winning pitcher **Barry Zito** of the Oakland A's are both alumni. The **Pigeon** is one of his key poses for pitchers, who drive off their back legs, generating power from their glutes and then land, jarringly, on the front leg, with the butt absorbing much of that repeated impact. "Their glutes get really tight right after they pitch," Jaeger says. "So we have them do the Pigeon, holding it for 30 to 45 seconds, and that way they don't get nearly as sore."

Real Men Don't: If you have a knee injury or chronic soreness there, skip this one. If that's you, or if you just find this very tough, use the gentler **Pigeon Variation** that follows. That's the one we'll be doing in our first, easier workout at the end of the book.

THE PIGEON

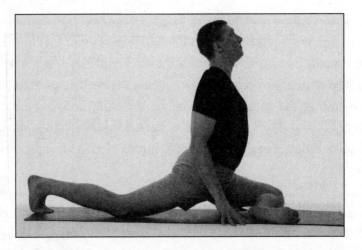

◆ Get on all fours. Swing your left leg out in front of you, bend it to a right angle at the knee, and place it side-down on the floor. Your left foot is near the right hand (see photo).

◆ Kick the right leg back and straight, keeping the torso upright. Try to keep that right hip as close as you can to the ground. Support yourself with your hands and arms on either side of you (you may need to be on your fingertips) alongside your chest. Hold your trunk upright—think of a pigeon with its chest puffed out and its little arms down. Long about now, you should be feeling a strong stretch in the outside of your left butt.

◆ Inhaling, draw yourself even more upright, chest and head higher, then exhale and lean forward, folding your upper body down and resting it on the bent left leg (if you can). Slide the hands and arms as far forward as they will go on the floor in front of you.

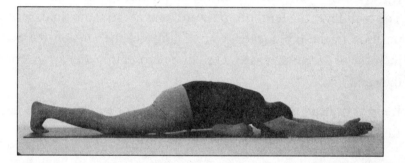

To do this part, at first you may have to bend the left knee more than 90 degrees, placing the calf on the floor closer to the thigh. As you get more flexible, you will gradually be able to straighten it so that it approaches a right angle with the thigh. Adjust as you can.

◆ Stay with it. This can be uncomfortable at first; breathe deeply (as always, through the nose). Better yet, as you inhale, imagine yourself sending the oxygen to the areas that are feeling this self-inflicted emergency the worst. If nothing else, it will distract you from any discomfort in your left leg and hip. You should also be feeling a strong stretch in your right groin at this point. But it's all good! You're opening up those ultra-tight areas.

◆ Hold for 8 full breaths if you can. To release, inhale and push yourself back up with your arms.

◆ Rest a bit, then reverse the legs. Okay, you're done. The **Pigeon** has landed.

PIGEON ALTERNATE

◆ Lie on your back with both knees bent, feet flat on the floor. Lift up the left foot and turn the leg so you can place your left ankle— the outside edge—on your right thigh, just above the knee.

◆ Then reach through your bent left leg with both hands, lifting your right leg so you can grasp it below the knee. Gently pull your right leg in toward your chest with the ankle still in place on the knee. This will lever the left knee outward, and at the same time, shift its position in the hip socket. You should feel the tension there and increase or decrease it as you see fit by loosening your arms around the right leg.

◆ Keep your head on the ground; don't strain or reach with the neck. Repeat on the other side.

The Mini-Workout: Now you've got 10 poses (for upper- and lower-body flexibility) to practice as we continue to work our way up to the full routines. Using the **Pigeon Alternate,** run through them together whenever you have time and/or before you try any of the new poses in chapters to come.

Yoga Jocks

SEAN BURKE

GOALTENDER, PHOENIX COYOTES

"I pretty much do yoga every single day, the majority of it at home with a videotape series by Bryan Kest that I really believe in. I'll always do at least a shortened version for about 20 to 25 minutes. On my days off, I step it up and do a more concentrated workout. If I miss a day, I start feeling guilty because it's almost like by not doing it, I'm only expecting average results out of myself. So needless to say, the days I take off are usually few and far between.

"I have to tell you, that first class I went to, there were a bunch of elderly women in the class, and they were so flexible, I thought for sure I was going to be completely embarrassed. I was dripping with sweat, and these ladies just breezed through the class. I thought, 'This isn't right.'

"Initially, there were poses I couldn't quite master, probably because I'm so big. But really, everybody goes through that in the beginning. As you get better and more familiar and dedicate yourself, it gets so much better, and before you know it, you're amazed at the benefits you get from yoga."

CHAPTER 5

Yoga Power: Building Functional Strength & Muscle Energy

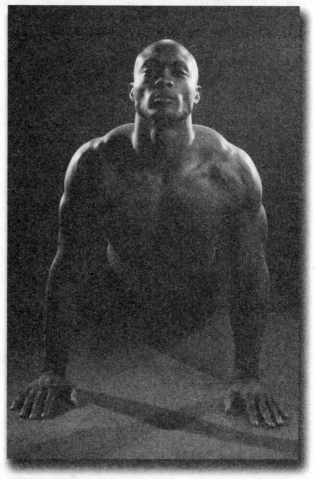

©Rob Lindsay 2003

Eddie George, Heisman Trophy winner and star NFL running back, says, "Yoga definitely builds strength. I've noticed it mostly in my upper body—there's an extra endurance factor."

Flexibility is yoga's main course, the dish that brings everyone to the table. You'll find out, though, that there's a lot more to the meal. Probably the biggest surprise for guys who try yoga is that the flexibility entrée comes with an extra helping—a side order of serious strength training (on the house). And that goes for both ordinary Joes and zillionaire athletes.

"I got into yoga thinking it was all about flexibility," says Dan Levitan, 48, a piano technician living in Brooklyn, New York. "But I found out that my concept of it was much too narrow." He started practicing nine years ago to compensate for the demands of his profession—it's hard physical work. "We get a lot of back trouble, tendonitis, carpal tunnel," Dan says. "Basically, I didn't want to end up looking like the old-timers I saw around me." But as he did more yoga he found that "Your body really gets stronger. Not bulky, but powerful. Your muscles are just charged with energy, which I really love."

Even **Eddie George,** who's so strong he's been on the cover of *Muscle & Fitness* magazine, went into yoga for flexibility and came out with more power, too. "It definitely builds strength," he says. "I've noticed that mostly in the upper body." Remember, this is a guy who bench-presses 400 pounds and squats about 500, according to Titans' strength and conditioning coach Steve Watterson.

In a study published in 2001, University of California at Davis scientists tested volunteers before and after eight weeks of twice-weekly yoga sessions. After that short time they found that "isokinetic muscular strength for elbow extension and elbow flexion and knee extension increased 31, 19 and 28 percent, whereas isometric muscular endurance for knee flexion increased 57 percent." (Flexibility and oxygen intake shot up, too.) As Ezra Amsterdam, one of the researchers on the study, put it, those are "pretty remarkable improvements."

Some of those gains come from improved flexibility and greater range of motion, as we discussed earlier. But yoga also generates its own unique kind of power.

Yoga strength is a tensile strength, born of holding sustained poses and using your own body weight as dynamic, living resistance. When you stay in a challenging yoga pose for, say, 10 breaths or 30 seconds, you are stressing those muscles for a much longer time than it takes to curl a dumbbell or perform some other kind of rep (how long's that take, maybe a second?). "Weight-lifting is a ballistic motion," says Craig Aaron, a yoga trainer in Atlanta, "while yoga is more about sustained strength training." As Eddie George puts it: "It's an endurance thing."

While weight-lifting builds bulk, it also shortens and tightens muscles. Yoga lengthens them, generating strength throughout the entire range of motion. (Yoga and pumping iron actually work really well together; see sidebar later in this chapter.) Rather than isolating muscles the way Cybex or Nautilus machines do, yoga moves recruit muscle groups from all over your body. These factors combined give yoga strength training one huge advantage: It builds functional strength, real-world power for real-world tasks.

Coach Watterson sees this in George. "Eddie's not just weight-room strong," Watterson says. "He's really a powerful guy, well balanced and flexible, strong in ways that help him perform as an athlete."

Most of us don't need NFL muscles, but we all need functional strength. What else is it good for? Well, the first use for anyone's muscles is supporting your skeletal system in the proper position. When that support and alignment are there, everything, even your internal organs, works as it should. And muscle strength helps maintain bone density for men as well as women. Beyond that—and beyond looking good on the beach—the main benefit of increased strength is to help you do things better. That is a) better than you otherwise would and b) better than the other guy. Including sports.

You can see functional strength triumph in any yoga class. Nick Cardillicchio, a 35-year-old New York photographer who goes to four classes a week, has noticed that "You see tiny women there that can do handstands but you'll see men with big muscles that can't do them." To him, that means that "in yoga you build strength, but you also learn to use it more effectively."

Men, you won't muscle up or get big from yoga like you do from lifting; odds are, you'll just look really toned. But underneath, invisibly, you'll be stronger and you'll greatly increase your muscle stamina. You can see the difference in the body types that each exercise produces. "Instead of the cannonball body-builder look," Aaron says, "really strong yogis look like strong rope, they have a kind of braided cable tensile strength."

This super-toning is part of why those women in yoga classes look so darn good—they're ripped, but in a pleasing, yoga-firm way. As Nick Cardillicchio says, "You can bounce a quarter off some of the girls in these classes." Not that we recommend that, you understand; the guy's just making a point.

Another remarkable improvement over traditional strength-training (weights, pushups, etc.) is how much more attention and awareness yoga demands. Instead of simply pushing or lifting *something else* as hard as you can, you have to maintain total control of the weight and the weight-lifter—both of which are you. You're exerting like crazy, but at the same time you're also maintaining your balance, noticing and correcting tiny movements, compensating, making adjustments, regulating your breathing. . . . This makes yoga strength-training much more complex and much more demanding mentally than just pushing plates. No autopilot here—you've got to concentrate and bear down, alert and awake, or it just won't happen.

Don't worry, though, you can still feel the burn without the iron. As you'll see very soon, these strength poses are intense. And by simply holding them longer you can rachet the difficulty right up there—your manhood will be tested.

We'll start by practicing strength poses that emphasize the lower body, then the upper body and finally a couple of killer poses that challenge your muscles head-to-toe.

LEGS AND LOWER BODY

THE WARRIOR (OR WARRIOR I)

This is one of the great all-around yoga moves, but I especially like it for the intense leg work involved, which you'll feel from butt to ankle. While it's toning leg muscle, the **Warrior** also stretches the pecs, the sides of the chest and the upper back. And as you'll see, there's a little bit of a balance challenge, too.

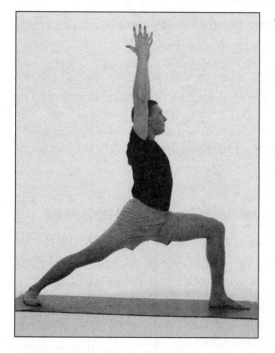

◆ Stand with your feet about 4 or 4½ feet apart. Now turn your right foot in slightly; you're going to use that puppy as an anchor.

◆ Turn the left foot out, forming as close to a 90-degree angle with the side of your body as possible. (If you can't do this at first, work up to it.) The front heel should be in line with the arch of the back foot.

◆ Inhale and raise your arms, extending them overhead, roughly alongside the ears.

◆ Now rotate your torso and head—the whole upper half—to the left, squaring your shoulders and aligning your gaze the same way the left foot is facing.

◆ Exhale as you bend your left leg at the knee, so the knee is directly over the ankle, shin perpendicular to the floor. Your weight and upper body will move forward, too; you should start feeling the stress in your left leg. But don't lean or tilt forward over the knee—keep the torso erect, eyes and head up.

◆ Check the back foot and make sure it's dug into the mat; the whole back leg should be engaged and alive with muscle energy.

◆ The arms are extended high, but you're not going for a big stretch here; keep your shoulder blades down in their normal resting place. The neck, throat and jaw are relaxed.

◆ Hold this for 10 complete breaths: 5 deliberate inhales, then exhales through the nose (roughly 30 seconds).

◆ Inhale and come up, straightening the left leg, moving your body back to a centered stance. Turn the feet and the torso back so you're facing front again.

◆ Rest, then reverse the feet and repeat, facing the other way, turning the right foot out.

Tip: The more you bend the front knee and lower yourself, the harder the workout for that leg. Think of martial arts guys crouching in their *katas*—that's how you want your stance to be in the **Warrior.** But your front knee shouldn't extend out past the ankle; if that happens, widen your stance.

WARRIOR II

Try this variation; in the next chapter, we'll learn **Warrior III.**

◆ Assume the stance as in **Warrior I** and bend the front leg the same way. Remember, both legs are active.

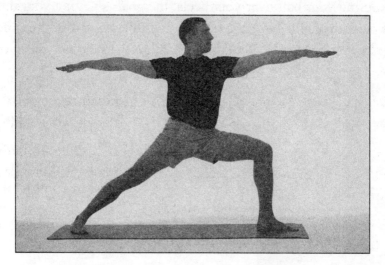

◆ Instead of raising your arms overhead, just lift them up from your sides and extend them out horizontally. And this time don't turn your whole upper body toward the front foot; just turn your head and look out over your extended left arm and hand.

◆ Stretch your arms out away from each other. Hold for 10 breaths.

◆ Repeat the opposite way (other leg bent; looking in that direction).

While **Warrior** feels natural and even sort of macho, the **Chair** is one of those awkward-feeling, difficult yoga positions for most guys. The tendency you have to fight is pitching the torso forward. Try to keep your lower back and torso vertical while you squat and lower down into the imaginary chair. Like any squatting exercise, this gives you a hard-core legs and butt workout, plus your shoulders and chest get stretched.

THE CHAIR

◆ Standing with feet 6 inches or so apart, inhale and raise your arms overhead, putting your palms together.

◆ Exhale and bend your knees, squatting straight downward and lowering your butt over your heels; the goal is getting your thighs as close to parallel with the floor as possible. As you go down, look up at your hands.

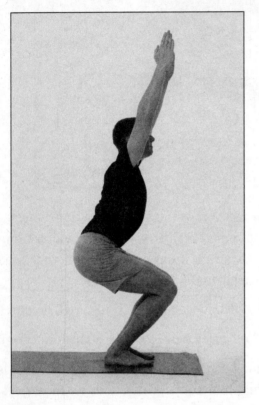

♦ Breathe and try to get lower—consciously try to tuck your tailbone down and under your butt. Keep the arms up high and don't let them pitch forward; they should be in line with your ears.

♦ Hold this position for 10 full breaths.

♦ Inhale and straighten the knees, lifting also with the arms. Exhale and drop arms to your sides.

♦ Repeat twice more.

UPPER BODY

Front Plank and Side Plank

These poses are so-named because they ask you to hold your entire body straight as a board. While doing that you're also going to be supporting all your body weight with fewer limbs than usual (heh-heh). Doing this not only strengthens your arms and upper body, but also gives you an extra dimension—the combination of strength-training with balance work—that makes yoga uniquely challenging.

Another great thing about these **Planks** is that they're completely symmetrical. If you're bench-pressing, for example, you can cheat unconsciously; your strong side will sometimes do more than its share of the work. But since the **Planks** work one arm at a time, each has to take all the weight individually—and thus, equally.

Keep in mind: Holding our bodies stiffly like this seems to make us want to stop breathing. Keep the breath flowing. To help you do that, we'll time the exercises by counting breaths.

FRONT PLANK

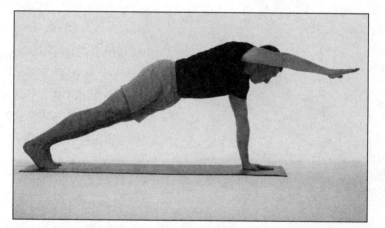

◆ Start in a pushup position, with the torso raised, shoulders over the wrists. Stretch the fingers wide on both hands, giving yourself a bigger, active platform on which to place your weight. Your body's a straight line from heels to head.

◆ Shift your body weight over a little to the left so that arm—extended but not locked at the elbow—is now supporting you, and extend your right arm straight out in front of you, palm down. Look down or at your right fingertips.

◆ Hold for 5 slow breaths, then return to both arms.

◆ Rest for a few breaths, then repeat on the other side. Do 3 reps on each arm.

Note: If you can't do this pose at first, just alternate shifting the weight from one arm to the other without taking either one off the floor.

SIDE PLANK

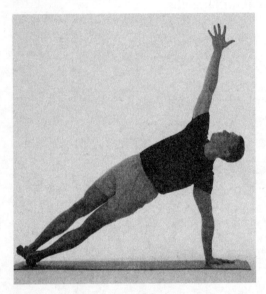

This one takes the balance challenge up a notch. Lose concentration here and you will fall on your Real Man's butt. You also need to fight the impulse to sink down into what feels like a safer position. Extend yourself up and out—go for it!—into a more precarious pose.

◆ In the starting pushup position, shift your weight onto the left arm as before. But this time, take the right arm out to the side, then turn your whole body up and to the right. You are now sideways to the floor instead of facing it, with all the weight on your left arm. Look up toward the ceiling at your right hand. Both arms form a straight line with each other.

◆ Now take your right foot slightly off the ground and rest it on the left foot that's on the floor. The two feet are now ankle-to-ankle. This can put your body into sway; you're now balancing your entire body—and holding all your body weight—on your left hand and the side of your left foot.

◆ Here comes the second balance test: Raise your hips and mid-section higher up, away from the floor. Get as high as you can, then find your equilibrium there. Your body's straight like a plank again, but now the board is sideways.

◆ Hold for 5 breaths, then gently swing back down to a two-arm pushup, or come down on your hands and knees.

◆ Rest briefly and then repeat on other side.

TOTAL BODY

We've done the lower body, we did the upper, now it's time to strengthen the entire package. Here are two very intense strength-building moves that you'll feel pretty acutely in the upper body, but which actually work every muscle fiber from toes to scalp.

I'm calling the first one the **Killer Yoga Pushup;** in yoga classes you'll hear it referred to as *Chatarunga*. The second one, the **Wheel,** comes with a strenuous backbend. Just in case these two aren't tough enough for you, we'll show you how to super-charge them both for a truly *sick* strength workout.

KILLER YOGA PUSHUP

◆ Get in the starting **Plank** or pushup position. Tuck your tailbone down and under to maintain the straight line of your body; you don't want your butt sticking up. Elbows are in, close to the sides of your chest.

◆ Exhale and slowly lower your torso and legs till you're 2 inches off the mat, like you are toward the beginning or end of a regular pushup. But unlike a pushup, you want to:

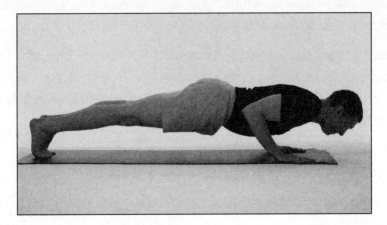

◆ Hold it right there. Don't tense the neck or raise the head; just keep looking down at the floor. As the strain increases—your arms may get shaky—concentrate on breathing smoothly and deeply. If nothing else, it will take your mind off what a beating your arms and pecs are taking.

◆ Keep the thighs and the front of the calves strong and engaged (you may find that you've recruited these muscles automatically to help hold yourself up). If you don't, you'll lose the straight line and your legs will slump to the floor.

◆ Hold for 10 full breaths. On an exhale, release your body down to the floor.

◆ Rest briefly, then repeat 2 more times.

═══════════ SUPER-CHARGE IT! ═══════════

If you want to be even more macho about it, try this: Instead of maintaining the weight on the toes and balls of your feet, roll the feet over onto their front sides (soles up). This will shift your torso forward a little, so your hands are planted further below the shoulders than before. Now slowly shift the position of your feet back so you're on your toes, which will slide you backward to the original position. Using just the motion of your feet to move yourself, go back and forth three times. This will make the **Killer Yoga Pushup** even more deadly.

THE WHEEL

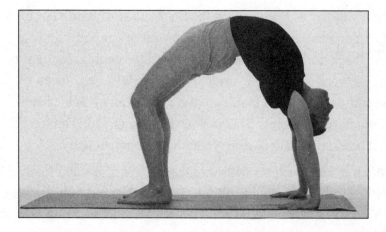

This one is really wild. It bends your entire body backward in a rounded wheel shape. Unless you're a gymnast or a cheerleader who does backflips, this is something you've probably never experienced in your life. So you're in foreign territory here and the natives are hostile. But hey, we're manly men, right?

Your legs will get a great workout as well as your arms, while you're stretching the chest and other muscles on your front—and flexing and strengthening the spine big-time. Because your head and neck are exposed and vulnerable, be very careful and make sure your footing and grip with your feet and hands is secure. For me, this pose is exhausting while doing it, but strangely energizing a short time afterward. See if it recharges you, too.

◆ Lie on your back with your arms and legs extended. Bend your knees and place your feet soles-down on the floor about where your knees were. If you can reach out and grab your ankles, that's about right.

◆ Exhale and push your tailbone and butt up off the floor. Your weight is now on your feet and the tops of your shoulders.

◆ Keeping the legs as they are, lift both arms off the floor, bend the elbows tightly and place the hands down on either side of your head, with the fingers pointing back toward the rest of your body (backwards, in a sense).

◆ Push your arms down against the floor and slowly lift your back off the floor a few inches. As your raise your upper body, let your head drop back down, raising the chin toward the ceiling, so the very top of the head grazes the floor. Now *carefully* rest more of your weight on your head. Don't put too much weight on the head—you could hurt your neck. This is your launching pad: The feet, hands and head are all supporting your slightly arched body.

◆ On an exhale push up with your hands and arms, and really drive with your legs, extending all four limbs as far and fully as you can. This will raise your head off the floor; just let it gently fall back. Your lower and upper body is stretched into a circular shape (but the hands and feet are still a few feet apart; the circle isn't closed) and all areas are humming with energy and effort. Breathe!

◆ Maintain the effort and the position for 5 full breaths if you can.

◆ When you feel you need to come down, exhale and start tilting the head back up (like you're nodding it yes), engaging the neck muscles so that when you lower yourself, the back of the head— not the top—will contact the floor. As the head moves out of the way, slowly lower yourself downward by bending all four of your "legs" evenly, letting your whole back body settle to the floor. Come down slow, don't drop.

◆ Rest and repeat 2 more times.

SUPER-CHARGE IT!

Take your time and get full control of yourself in the **Wheel** over a few weeks or months. Then make it even tougher by extending fully as described above, and doing pushups by lowering and raising your upper body with your arms. The legs stay strong but don't change their position. Gimme five. Now *that's* hard. As Michael, who devised this torture, says: "You ain't lived until you've done this."

EAST MEETS WEST: YOGA + PUMPING IRON

To lots of traditional yoga folks, lifting weights is a symbol of everything they don't like: a meat-eating, testosterone-laden, Western-aggression macho thing. But in our new-school, guy-yoga, cross-training way of doing things, it's not just okay to push some steel along with practicing yoga; it's actually a great idea. As the super-jocks of pro sports have found out, these two very different exercises complement each other really well. To steal a New Age term or two, yoga and pumping iron are symbiotic—they're practically Yin and Yang!

Truth is, there's nothing like lifting for building pure strength and especially muscle mass. But there are drawbacks to iron-pumping, including the risk of injury and getting that stiff, weight lifter's physique. The good news is that yoga's benefits counter those exact same problems. Yoga's strong where lifting's weak, if you will. That's good teamwork—something any red-blooded, sports-minded guy can understand.

- As we discussed earlier in this chapter, weights—especially weight machines like Cybex and Nautilus—isolate muscles to work them harder. Yoga recruits whole groups of muscles to work together. So you can build the muscles solo but also develop that integrated functional strength in your yoga workouts. Two kinds of strength is better than one, no?
- Iron pumping exercises tend to develop the big, exterior muscles like the pecs, biceps and quadriceps. Yoga hits all the little muscles, including stablizers in the core. So by doing both workouts, you're covering the entire waterfront.
- Lifting weights contracts muscles and leaves them tight, which can constrict your range of motion. But yoga lengthens the muscles, takes the tension out of them and restores the ROM. This in turn prepares the muscles to be contracted fully and efficiently the next time.
- Weight-training actually tears muscles, creating scar tissue (that's what forms the visible bulk). Yoga can't repair all the damage, but putting the flexibility back into the muscles creates better blood flow and circulation, bringing oxygen that helps those muscles heal. Dr. Craig Aaron, the Atlanta yoga teacher who works with Georgia Tech's athletic teams, says that "doing yoga on non-weight-lifting days definitely helps you rehab and recover."
- After you're done lifting, the stress creates a caustic by-product, lactic acid. Again, yoga to the rescue. As Dr. Aaron explains it, "The deep yoga stretches wring the lactic acid and other inflammatory chemicals right out of there."

Ever watch pro wrestling on TV, such as the WWE (formerly the WWF)? If so, you will probably recognize Diamond Dallas Page. He started doing yoga after hurting his back about 3 to 4 years ago and recently retired at age 46 (he's trying to become an actor). But he's still doing yoga and he's still weight-training. Only Dallas has combined yoga and weight training in his own unique way—he does them both in the same workout.

"Every day I do at least 30 minutes of yoga," he says. "Most times an hour. And sometimes I'll take a class for an hour and a half. But I literally incorporated it into my training. I'll be in Gold's Gym in Hollywood and in between sets I'm doing Ashtanga power positions, and I don't care who's watching me."

Sounds good. Make you wonder, though, how did those other guys on the pro wrestling circuit react to Dallas doing yoga? "Oh man," he says. "Guys busted my chops in wrestling big-time. But I couldn't care less what they thought. And one by one, guys who had injuries or physical problems would come up to me and start asking me questions. And I turned some of them onto it, too."

CHAPTER 6
Balance & Body Control

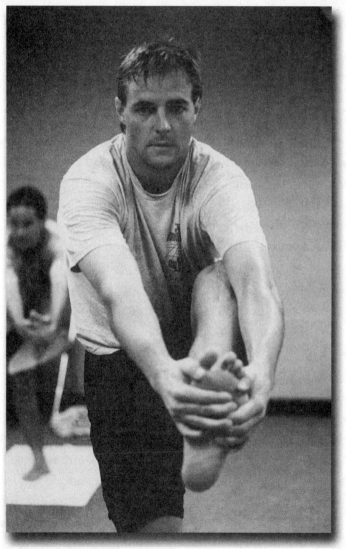

®Heather Selwitz/*Palm Beach Post*

New York Mets pitching ace Al Leiter gets ready to stretch out in a one-legged balance pose. He's been practicing since 1990 and says, "Yoga's one of the hardest workouts I've ever done. It's awesome, absolutely the best."

For sheer fun, working on your balance has got to be the best part of yoga. I think you're really going to enjoy it, even though you'll probably keel over a few times. But you know what? Trying to keep your balance, feeling yourself wavering and teetering, then when you know you can't stay up any longer, finally giving in and falling down is its own goofy kind of fun—kinda like when we were kids.

At the same time, balance work is also one of the most challenging aspects of yoga, and these moves are some of the toughest to master. The upside of this high degree of difficulty is that after you've worked on these positions for a while (and yes, bounced off the mat a few times) and you start to see your balance and body control really improving, you'll feel that you've made real athletic progress. And you'll be right.

Keep in mind, though, that the benefits don't end with being able to stay up on your toes like a dancer, or maintain some other esoteric position. As with strength, the goal is not just to *have* good balance, but to do something with it. Call it functional balance. **Joe Inman,** a yoga devotee who plays on the PGA Senior Tour, explains what good balance allows you to do, in his game or any other. "Whether you're a pitcher in baseball or tackling someone in football," he says, "you can't *deliver energy* without balance. It's the same in golf: If you're falling around this way and that way, you can't make contact with the ball the same way every time like you need to do."

In golf, no one's trying to knock you over (hopefully). However, balance is big in power games like football, too, and not just for the "skill players." Down in the NFL trenches, for example, it looks like those linemen just go after each other with brute strength. But 6'5", 275-pound Denver Broncos defensive end **Lester Archambeau** improved his balance and agility through yoga—and he says those are equally important weapons for a hulking guy like him. "We always have our weight shifting," he told the *Rocky Mountain News* back in 2000 (he's since retired). "Believe it or not, we often play on one foot, not two. You've got to have body control."

Another great thing about balance poses is how they force you to develop your focus and concentration. Since you really don't want to fall over, my guess is you'll be paying attention. As you've already seen, almost every standing pose requires maintaining your equilibrium in some way, and in this chapter you'll learn five new positions that are *primarily* balance challenges.

Real Men Don't: Hold their breath. You may find yourself focusing so intently on maintaining your precarious position(s) that you stop breathing, trying to remain totally still. Don't geek up. That's what Denver yoga guru Danny Poole calls it: "Everyone is so worried about losing their balance that they start holding their breath and grimacing," he says, talking about his pupils on the University of Colorado football team and the Denver Broncos. "So I come over and tell 'em, 'Soften the face and breathe, soften the face and breathe. . . .'"

TREE

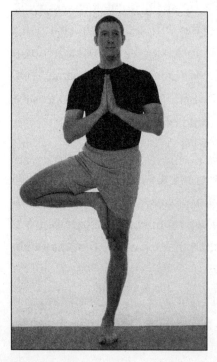

The **Tree** is an excellent way to get started; it's very simple, but at the same time, not. When learning this and other standing balance poses, you can start standing within arm's length of a wall and use it when necessary to keep yourself upright. As you get more proficient, move away from the wall. Another hint: If you've got pants or shorts with a slippery surface, your foot'll slide down and off in this pose. Try something made of grippier material—regular cotton sweatpant material isn't bad, but the synthetic stuff doesn't work as well. Alternatives: Yank the leg of your shorts up a little and go skin to skin, or take your sticky mat and put it between your thigh and foot to get a good grip.

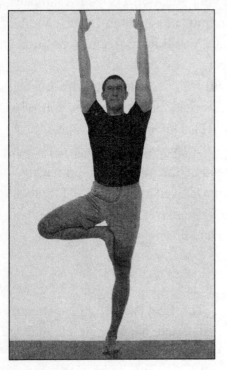

◆ Stand up barefoot, so you can grip the floor or mat better. Now shift your weight to your left foot. With your right foot still on the floor, really ground yourself on your left foot. Think about the "four corners" of your foot: the inside and outside edges and the heel and ball. You want your weight distributed equally between those four points of support.

◆ Bend the right knee, keeping the left one straight (but don't lock the knee). Reach down with either or both hands (this is where you can lean one arm against the wall if need be) and take hold of your right ankle.

◆ Raise the foot up, turning the right knee outward as you do, and place the sole of the foot flat against the inside of the left thigh, as high up as you can go. Ideally, your toes are pointing straight down at the floor, but any way you can keep that puppy up there is great. Digging the heel in a little more than the rest of the foot may help you keep it in place.

◆ Let go of the right foot and stand erect with the knee sticking out at as close to a right angle to the left, straight leg as possible. The foot and leg are pressing firmly against each other; you want some tension between them. Take a few slow breaths.

◆ Now slowly lift your arms and place your palms together, prayer-style, with the thumbs resting against the middle front of your chest. Keep the balancing leg charged and active. Take a few more breaths. Try to stay balanced for 30 seconds.

◆ Now raise your arms over your head as if you're a referee signaling for a touchdown (the same way you held them in **Warrior I**). Keep the arms raised for another 15 seconds.

◆ Lower the arms and drop them down to your sides. Release the right foot and let it down to the ground.

◆ Rest, then ground the right foot the same way. Repeat the exercise with the left leg raised.

Tip: To help maintain balancing poses, pick a spot in the middle distance—a point on a wall, for example, if you're standing in the middle of a room—and keep your gaze concentrated on that point.

THE EAGLE

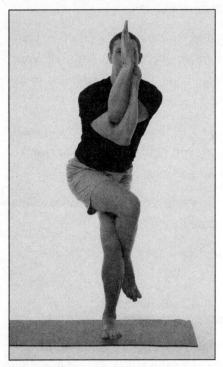

We did the top half of this pose to stretch out the back muscles in the chapter on upper body flexibility. Here we'll use the lower body to put a tricky twist on the **Tree.** If this is really tough—you can see that even our model has trouble standing completely upright—don't worry about it. Just do the **Tree** and the others. But it's definitely worth a try.

◆ Standing up, bend your knees, keeping your heels on the floor. Grounding yourself firmly on your left foot, lift your right leg and cross it over in front of the left. Now wrap the lower right leg around the left calf so your legs are intertwined (see picture). Squeeze your thighs together and try to square your hips so they face straight out in front of you.

◆ Keep the legs where they are and maintain your balance. Now you want to do the same thing with your forearms, as we did before. Bend both your arms at the elbow in front of you and place the left elbow inside the bend of the right one. Snake the right forearm around and behind the left forearm so they look braided together. Press your right fingers against your left palm, both hands pointing straight up. Try to stand as straight as possible. Lifting the head will help.

◆ You've got it, now just hold it. Breathe evenly and slowly, concentrating on that point in the near distance to help you keep balanced. Hold for 30 seconds if you can.

◆ Unwrap, come down to the mat and shake your limbs out to loosen them. Then do the exercise in reverse.

SUPER-CHARGE IT!

Making any balance pose more challenging is simple: Just close your eyes. But be warned, this makes things a whole lot more difficult.

We having fun yet? Good. Now let's give the legs a rest and take the balance challenge to the arms.

THE CROW

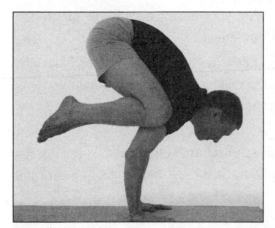

This a really nifty move that looks impossible when you first see someone else doing it (you can see here how it resembles a perched bird). But when you get into it, it rapidly narrows to a few points of concentration. That doesn't necessarily make it any easier. For one thing, it's a helluva triceps, arms and wrists workout, in addition to the balance work.

There's a greater fear factor in the **Crow** than with the standing poses, as you risk tipping forward onto your face. Approach it carefully, and odds are you will almost always tip backwards instead. However, you might feel better putting a big pillow or cushion in front of you at first to catch your fall—no face-plants!

◆ Squat down on your mat, opening your legs out to the side as you lower so the knees are wider than the hips. Lean forward and reach your arms out between your legs to place your hands on the mat in front of you, shoulder-width apart. Establish your base by spreading the palms and fingers as wide as possible with the index fingers pointing straight ahead. Come up on the balls of your feet.

◆ Lean forward a little more, putting more weight on the hands. Raise up on your toes, tilting forward even more. Elbows are bent, your arms are supporting you, and your triceps are under the insides of your knees/thighs. Here comes the tricky part.

◆ Lift one foot off the ground and let the back of the upper arm on that side take the weight of the leg. Now you're a tripod.

◆ When you feel ready, take the other foot off the ground and balance totally on your two hands and arms. The insides of your knees are supported by the triceps. With your head basically parallel to the floor, look down squarely at the mat.

◆ Hold for 5 to 10 breaths, as many as you can. As you perch or roost here, you'll probably have to make some mini-adjustments to stay balanced; try to make them as tiny and deliberate as possible so the motion doesn't tip the bird.

◆ Rock back onto your heels and return to the squat, releasing the arms to come up off the floor. Shake out the wrists before doing the pose again.

This may take a few tries, but when you get it, you'll feel like an Olympic gymnast! Give yourself a perfect 10.

Tip: If you're having difficulty getting set in this pose, try starting by squatting with your heels on a block or a thick phone book to start. This will lessen the distance you travel as you lean forward into the pose.

Moving back to leg-land, let's try a standing balance that's called **Warrior III** by some folks and known as **Airplane** by others. I guess the straight leg is the landing gear or something. Anyway, this is a good one to move into right out of **Warrior II** or straight from the **Tree.** (Like those poses, it's a real leg strengthener.)

WARRIOR III

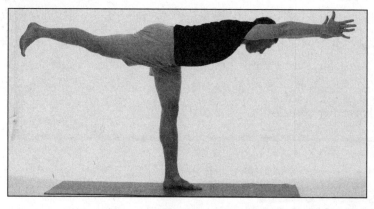

◆ Standing on your mat, bend both knees slightly, then reach down and put both your hands on your left knee.

◆ Exhale and, keeping the left leg slightly bent, raise your right leg and extend it straight out behind you. As you do this, also pitch your head and torso forward so your leg, torso and head all form a straight line parallel to the floor. Back is straight. Breathe.

◆ Now push up and straighten the left leg. Your leg and torso are at right angles. As you straighten, your hands will naturally come off the left knee. Extend your arms straight out in front of you. Your attention is now going to naturally move to your balance and the supporting leg, but don't forget the back leg. Keep it engaged and straight.

◆ Hold like this for 10 full breaths. Gaze steadily at the floor through-out, keeping both back and legs straight (but don't lock the left knee).

◆ Either inhale and come down on both feet or try reaching the arms out to the sides in airplane style (they're the wings). Then rock backward onto both feet again.

◆ Rest and repeat on the other leg.

Tip: To make this easier, start by placing a sturdy high-backed chair about 3 feet in front of you. Lean forward and hold onto the top of it with both hands. Then, as you raise the back leg and lean forward more, the chair will keep you stable. Then let go and begin to balance, reaching downward and extending your arms together as we described. Grab the chair as needed. Then as you get more comfortable, leave the chair out of it and fly solo.

DEEP THOUGHTS

I hope you had fun testing and improving your balance; as I said, it's one of my favorite parts of practicing yoga. But it was hard. Let's face it: At first, you probably sucked, am I right?

But that's good, too. Confronting our lack of proficiency here can offer a little lesson in humility. Let's say you go to a class, and you're falling over; you can't hold your balance in some tricky pose. Not only that, but then you look around and see that other folks in the class, including women and guys who you didn't think looked very athletic, are holding themselves steady like some Rocks of Gibraltar. Well, it's humbling. And that's a good thing, every once in a while, to get a reminder that a) You don't know everything b) You can't do everything and c) Some people are better than you are at some things. Plus d) It never pays to make assumptions about other people.

Okay, end of sermon. Don't know what came over me. Let's get back to jock talk.

BALANCE & STRENGTH-TRAINING

When you were doing the strength poses like **Side Plank** in the last chapter, I'm sure you felt the balance challenges involved. Likewise, while you were doing the balance poses in this chapter, I'm absolutely positive you realized they require *tons* of strength and muscular exertion. This dual aspect is a very important way in which yoga strength-training is more challenging and rewarding than other kinds of workouts.

Often these poses require you to handle your body weight and balance yourself with fewer and smaller body parts than you normally do. Like in **Crow,** for example, all your weight and the entire balance burden are on your arms and hands. It's like every one of these exercises is Super-Charged. Even more important, working on both aspects *simultaneously* compounds the stress, making both the strength and the balance workouts much more difficult.

Eric Hiljus, a right-handed starting pitcher for the Oakland A's, is really high on this part of his yoga training. He's been working with California teacher Alan Jaeger since 1991, and he's been amazed, first of all, at how much "Yoga does create strength. I don't do nearly as much yoga during the baseball season as in the off-season," explains the 30-year-old. "It's really hard with our long days and the travel. But if I was able to do yoga all year long, I would definitely not have to lift a weight. *I wouldn't touch a weight.* And when I do start lifting weights in spring training—after not lifting all winter, but doing yoga—it's like I never even stopped."

Hiljus is a big guy: 6'6", 240. He's got big muscles to work. Yoga can challenge a guy his size, he believes, due to that super-stressful combo of balance and strength work. "To get a sense of how hard it is," he says, "think of a pushup. If you do one, it's not that hard at all. But if you took a medicine ball and you balanced on that with both hands and tried to do your pushup on that, it's like 20 times harder. That's because now not only are you picking up that weight, but you're also balancing that weight. That's what will help you get your strength."

The one-legged poses like **Warrior III** are a real bear for him, Hiljus reports. "When you have to lean forward and balance on that one leg, not only are you creating balance, but now you're creating strength because that one leg is holding all your weight while it's balancing your entire body."

Sounds kinda hard. But you're such a stud, you've already done all these toughies-but-goodies. Time to try something *really* challenging—like breathing.

Yoga Jocks

ROBBY GINEPRI

TENNIS PLAYER, ATP TOUR (TOP 100 RANKING)

When Ginepri, then 20, was having back pain, a fellow player at the 2001 U.S. Open told him about yoga.

"After the first class, I felt so relaxed, my whole body felt completely different—I was kinda surprised. I felt so relieved, and like all the toxins had been removed from my body.

"It definitely tones; you can tell it's a strength-builder. Plus, with more flexibility, your muscles stretch, your body isn't as tight, and that will help prevent injuries.

"For me, my groin area and hips are key. The balance work helps with all the side-to-side motion we do in tennis and your footwork. And the more you practice proper breathing in class, the more it will help you on the court; when you're in a tough match, that helps you to relax.

"Every time, as soon as I get out of class, I still feel great. I feel loose; it's great; it's almost feels like I'm floating."

CHAPTER 7
Cardio & Learning to Breathe (Again)

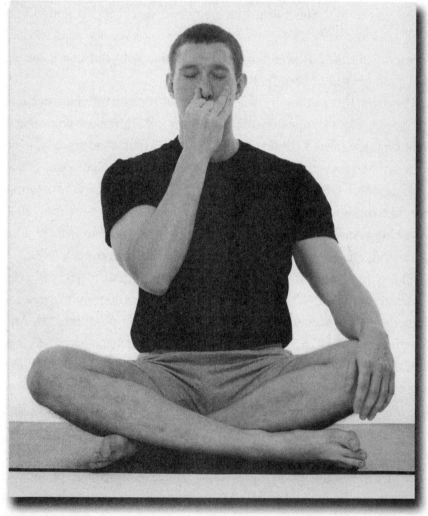

©Erica Berger, 2003

Alternate nostril breathing increases awareness of your breathing patterns and develops control over your respiration.

Lots of true believers will tell you that, on top of all the other great benefits yoga gives you, it's also a great cardiovascular workout. But I don't really buy that.

The **Sun Salute** we'll learn in chapter 10 will get the blood flowing; it's a nice warmup. I certainly agree with Mets pitcher **Al Leiter** and other fans of Bikram yoga (that's the 100-degree-room kind) that when you do it, "You sweat like crazy and your heart is pounding." And in some very fast-moving Ashtanga or Vinyasa yoga classes (sometimes called Power Yoga) you can also get your heart rate up and even get out of breath at times.

However I'm not totally sold on the hot-room treatment. For one thing, you can't duplicate it on your own, which makes you dependent on these heated studios to get your workouts. And frankly, even faster-moving yoga just ain't that big of a cardio challenge. Some yoga teachers are up front about that. "Honestly, is it a cardio workout, like running three miles? Even in the Asthanga style, I'd say no," says Craig Aaron. So to be Joe Jockman, you're going to want to continue with a solid cardiovascular practice, three workouts a week.

The way I figure it, for active guys a cardio goal in yoga is even counterproductive. What I mean by that is, we're coming to yoga for something new, something we don't already have in our arsenal. And to practice yoga in a jump-around-like-a-maniac, sweat-flying, breath-gasping, pulse-pounding way is defeating that purpose. We already have sports (and sex) for that. The added value here is learning how to move slowly, deliberately and consciously, in ways that improve body awareness and body control. Honestly, don't you have enough frantic activity in your life as it is?

Here's the clincher: By practicing yoga in the more traditional, slower way—using yogic breathing exercises—you will actually get some fantastic benefits, very similar to those you get from cardio work. Yoga achieves some of the same goals in very different ways— plus, it gives you a whole lot more. Yogic breath work will:

- *Increase oxygen intake*
- *Improve oxygen exchange (that's O molecules in, carbon dioxide or CO_2, out).*
- *Deepen your body awareness through focusing on the breath.*
- *Train and improve your focus and powers of concentration. And as we'll explore more fully later, these last two benefits are your tickets to The Zone, the realm of peak performance.*

To accomplish this, you'll have to rethink and revamp the way you're using your lungs and diaphragm. It also means trying a different kind of yoga work than we've done so far. We've been moving the whole body, stretching and bending—the stuff we normally think of as exercise. But breath work isn't like that, and trying to control the breath—making this unconscious process a conscious one—can be difficult. In a sense, it'll be:

LEARNING TO BREATHE
(ALL OVER AGAIN)

At this point, you may be wondering: Is this really necessary? After all, if you're reading this—in other words, you're not deceased—you're probably doing a pretty good job of breathing already. In fact, you do it around twenty thousand times a day. So how much work do you really need to do on that?

The fact is, most of us, including elite athletes, don't use anywhere near our total lung capacity. We barely use the diaphragm and belly to pump air in and out of our lungs, which is what they're designed for. Instead we're chest-breathers, taking quick, shallow breaths that don't fully expand and contract the bellows of our lungs. And because we get less air—and therefore less oxygen—that way, we have to take many more of these superficial "rabbit breaths" to get the job done.

You know your body needs oxygen in every cell and that the muscles and brain work better with more of that magic gas. But you still may not realize just how precious a commodity oxygen is. We take in about 17 fluid ounces of air with every inhale. However, that air only contains about 21 percent oxygen, and the air we breathe out contains about 16 percent—the remaining five is what we live on. That's a pretty narrow margin. Given that, you can see how increasing either the volume and/or that percentage would make a humongous change for the good.

Nobody breathes worse than a smoker, right? New York photographer Nick Cardillicchio says he "really smoked for 20 years, at least a pack a day. I'd wake up in the middle of the night, smoke, and go back to sleep." Then after September 11, he decided he had to quit the butts. "You have no idea how hard it is," he says. Four days into quitting he went to his first yoga basics class, and he's never lit up again. "It definitely kept me from smoking," Nick says. "You don't realize that you basically feel terrible all day long, you think it's normal. Then you do yoga and realize: 'I can feel like this?' I found out from yoga how much oxygen a person can get. The more oxygen you get, the more you're living."

Here's an even more drastic example. At a recent workshop Michael Lechonczak watched his teacher, John Friend, work with a New York City fireman whose lungs had been damaged in the World Trade Center attacks. After some gentle backbends and yogic breath work, the fireman got up on stage and said, "I've been to every doctor, every specialist, but I still had to retire—I couldn't breathe. This is the first time since September 11 that I've gone for 20 minutes without coughing."

Just by doing the yoga poses we've covered so far—before the breath work—you're already starting to get breathing benefits. In a study conducted at Ball State University (published in 2000), 287 college students took two 50-minute classes a week for 15 weeks. Then their lung capacity was remeasured and they showed an average 10 percent improvement. The reason, the scientists posited: "Yoga poses help increase lung capacity by improving flexibility in the rib area, shoulders and back, allowing the lungs to expand more fully.' This is especially helpful for those of us who do a lot of chest stuff at the gym and/or work at a computer, or both, which hampers the upper part of the lungs from taking a full breath.

After you learn to breathe better, these techniques will star) take hold in your subconscious, and eventually you will start us hem all the time. You may be amazed right away, though, to discc that your body is really up to, breathing-wise, and how much m(can do. It's like looking under your own hood while the motor is ing, then finding out about some higher-octane fuel that'll make i run even better.

BREATHING EXERCISES

To pump up the volume on our oxygen intake, we'll st rt with a very simple exercise called **Three-Part Breath.** For me, his was a real eye-opener—and a body opener. The day after I did this for the first time, my upper chest was sore just under my collarbones. It felt like I hadn't really expanded my uppermost chest in years and millions of breaths. Doing that seemed to break the locked-in rigidity; I never felt that pain again.

THREE-PART BREATH

You can do this one sitting in a chair or lying down. Remember, in all of these, as in the poses, breathe through the nose, not the mouth.

◆ Place your right hand on your belly, thumb above the navel and the rest of the hand below.

◆ Inhale slowly—maybe a slow 5-count—expanding the lower belly under your hand. Exhale, feeling the belly collapse. This is Part One.

◆ Part Two: Keep the right hand on your belly. Now place the left hand on your lower left ribcage—feel those bones under your palm, which is now stacked a little higher than the right hand. Inhale as before, but now, as your belly starts to feel full, simply . . . keep going. Draw more air into your nose until you start to feel the ribcage expand with the increased volume. To the 5-count of the belly-breath, add another 3 counts or so. (If you start with a different count, that's fine. Just go a few more beats.)

◆ Exhale slowly, feeling with your left hand—and following intently with your mind—how the ribcage settles back down and then, in sequence, the belly deflates as before. Repeat a few times and get comfortable.

◆ Part Three: Leave the right hand where it is and move your left hand higher up and toward the center of your chest, so the middle of your palm is around the breastbone and your fingers are at the base of your neck.

◆ Begin inhaling as before, into the belly, then into the ribs, then . . . go even further! Try adding another 3-count of inhalation to the Two-Part process—this is Part Three. Keep breathing in, filling up your upper torso so you feel the left hand move under the expanding chest and rising collarbones.

◆ Exhale slowly the same three-stage way, following the release of air from the upper chest, lower chest, ribs, upper abdomen and lower belly.

◆ Repeat 10 times.

See what a huge air-pumping station you can be if you try? Some experts estimate that we can take in as much as seven times as much air this way as in our normal shallow breathing. This is how you want to breathe when you're in the poses. You probably won't be able to open up as deeply—or pay this close attention—but that's the goal.

By breathing more deeply we also need to breathe less often, which creates a less-taxed, more relaxed metabolism. After all his yoga practice, Michael, the yoga consultant on this book, breathes so deeply that he only needs to take about six breaths a minute—that's less than ten thousand a day, or half the average guy's total. "When you breathe better, you can think more clearly," he reports. "And life becomes easier. Your body works better: the muscles, digestive system, the brain. . . ."

Clearly, more oxygen is better when it comes to sports performance. And even big-time athletes can do a lot better when it comes to their air intake. In fact, Colorado yoga trainer Danny Poole has seen in his work with football players that they often hold their breath at critical moments—the worst thing you could possibly do. As Poole says, "The body just freaks out when you hold your breath." Athletes with yoga training are more aware, so they can catch themselves holding their breath, Poole says. "If they can catch themselves in the first 10 seconds versus 20 seconds, that can make a big difference in sports. If the guy on the other side of the ball is holding his breath, you have an up on him."

But there's more to breathing than just the Big O. Your lungs must also carry out the vital process of "oxygen exchange." After they take oxygen in they need to get the waste gas carbon dioxide out. On the exhale you get rid of 100 times as much carbon dioxide as you inhale. Just as you can learn to take in more O, you can also learn to empty your lungs better—all the way to the bottom—and fully flush that CO_2. That's what this next exercise is all about.

POWER EXHALES

◆ Sit comfortably with your chest erect, either in a chair or cross-legged on a mat or the floor. Breathe normally through your nose. Belly is loose, in a neutral resting position.

◆ On the next exhale, snort the air vigorously out of your nose, as hard and fast as you can. You should really hear the wind rushing out of that narrow opening. At the same time, forcefully contract or draw your abdomen inward. You are literally compressing the bellows of your lungs to squeeze the older, stale air out of there. (You might want to have a tissue around in case any other old stuff comes flying out the nose hole.)

◆ Keep exhaling this way, ignoring the inhales. They will just happen naturally; let them be a passive motion and focus on contracting below and expelling air above.

◆ Do 25 times or as long as you can keep it up. Then do a second set.

━━━━━ SUPER-CHARGE IT! ━━━━━

Nancy Nielsen, a yoga teacher who's working with the NBA's Denver Nuggets, suggests this variation, done standing up. "As you inhale, bring your arms overhead. That brings more air down into the lower lobes of your lungs," she says. "Then on the forceful exhales, pull the arms vigorously down to your sides while bending them at the elbows and clenching your fists. Press your upper arms tightly against the sides of your rib cage as you bring them down, putting an even bigger squeeze on the lungs to empty them."

ALTERNATE NOSTRIL BREATHING

This next one might seem a little freaky, but I think it's worth experimenting with. If nothing else, it forces you to concentrate very closely on your breathing—and to control it. So you're building body control and practicing narrowing your focus.

As I said before, yoga traditionalists are fanatics about nose breathing. They believe that what you're inhaling this way is not just air, but *prana,* the energy or life force that sustains the universe. This is the yoga equivalent of *chi* in some other Eastern traditions (like tai chi).

Whatever. You can buy that or not. But even if you think of *prana* in our crude Western way, as simply oxygen, their nosy rationale makes a lot of sense. Using those two smaller cavities rather than the mouth, they say, properly regulates the amount and the pace of your breath, while the hairs and mucous membranes inside the nasal passages filter the air and heat it to the proper temp before it hits the rest of the body.

In his excellent book, *Body, Mind and Sport,* fitness expert John Douillard also makes the case that we are natural nose breathers. Look at newborns, he says, who basically only breathe through an open mouth when they are crying. And racehorses—as fast as they go and as great an effort as they make, breathe only through their noses. He has a whole program for training yourself to breathe nasally during sports competition—which he's used successfully with pro tennis players, triathletes and body builders, among others.

That's pretty advanced. For now, let's just go with the air flow and agree to breathe through the nose. Right now we'll breathe through one nostril and then the other. (Again, no one's watching, right?)

This technique (see the photo on page 75) is supposed to balance the activity in the two hemispheres of your brain (there's gotta be some major *prana* swimming around in there). In any case, lots of folks who try it say it does seem to calm them down and reduce any agitation they might bring to the mat with them. I've definitely noticed that at some times, but not at others. Give it a whirl, then rest for a few moments immediately afterward and see if you feel any different. As they used to say back in the '70s: If it feels good, do it. If not, get on with your life.

ALTERNATE NOSTRIL BREATHING

◆ Sit in a relaxed position, with your trunk upright enough for easy breathing.

◆ Reach up with your right thumb and close off your right nostril. Exhale through the left nostril.

◆ Now inhale slowly and deliberately through the left nostril. Stop when you feel your inhale is done. (For me, that's about a 6-count.)

◆ Use your finger or fingers to close off that left nostril. (Yoga purists insist that the ring and little fingers be used together for this; personally, I think you're old enough to decide for yourself.)

◆ Hold your breath with both nostrils closed for the same amount of time you inhaled.

◆ Now lift your thumb off the right nostril and exhale through it, for at least as long a count as you inhaled and then hold your breath. Longer is even better.

◆ At the end of the right-nostril exhale, inhale slowly through the same side, then hold both closed, then exhale through the left, etc.

◆ Repeat for a total of 20 cycles (from inhaling on one side to exhaling on that same side is one cycle).

If it distracts you to count, just time your breathing and holding by feel. As you get more comfortable, you may see your inhales, exhales and holds get longer. And don't squeeze the life out of your little nose; just apply enough pressure to do the job.

The Real Man

PETER SCIRIOS

ARCHITECT, 47, SAN LUIS OBISPO, CA

"I played semi-pro rugby for about seven years—and yoga was the result. I was having a lot of problems with my neck and my knees, and I was taking 6 to 8 ibuprofen a day. Yoga was purely therapeutic; I gradually got myself off the painkillers and I could walk normally again.

"When I got to my first class I was the only guy and I was thinking: *What am I doing here?* All these 40-year-old women were more flexible, and some even stronger than me, so it was very humbling.

"Finally, I gave up rugby and took up windsurfing as my adrenaline replacement. Again, I found yoga extremely helpful. The flexibility helped reduce the tightness after hours of sailing. And the incredible balance you develop you can use directly in windsurfing.

"I think yoga's allowed me to continue the things I enjoy—basketball, windsurfing, biking. I can keep up with guys 10 to 15 years younger than me. My body shape has changed drastically but I feel just as strong as I was. I have more endurance and weigh 30 pounds less.

"Also, I've been an architect for 20 years and I was struggling with the beginning of carpal tunnel syndrome from all the computer work and leaning over, and I have overcome that with yoga.

"I'm sold. I couldn't be what I am now if it wasn't for yoga."

CHAPTER 8

Working the Core:
Abs & Beyond

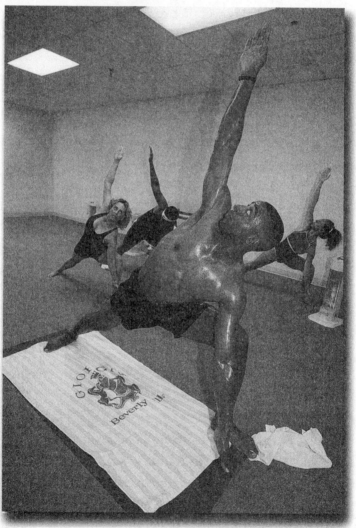

Bill Frakes/*Sports Illustrated*

Chris Carter, one of the best receivers in NFL history, in a Triangle variation. Renowned for the intensity of his conditioning program, he'd end his off-season training days with two hours of yoga.

O kay, I'm only going to say this once: You don't need rock-hard abs. In fact, that sharply defined "six pack" you see on models and magazine covers *isn't even something you really want.*

Think about it. In all the work we've done so far, we've seen how flexibility benefits you in so many ways and why *limber* strength gives you real functional power. In every area we've dealt with, that's the goal. So why, when it comes to the abdomen, would we suddenly covet big, prominent, *rigid* muscles?

We wouldn't. We don't. It's just as bad to have tight, contracted abs as it is to have any other muscle in that condition: It limits mobility and carries tension, which makes you more susceptible to injury. The six-pack just shows how overtrained and overdeveloped those specific muscles are, and as we've seen, symmetrical, overall development is the way to go.

Plus, very few of us even have the genetic ability to develop our abs to that extent, or to have them show. Most guys who aren't ab models have a couple inches of subcutaneous fat there and a normal skin thickness, both of which make it harder to see the definition. So the pursuit of the six-pack is really a losing game. Unclench that stomach. And you can stop holding your breath, too, which we tend to do when working and showing off our ab muscles.

Not to say that your ab muscles aren't important—they're crucial. In fact, this region of the body relies more on muscle than almost any other. There's no supporting bone structure around the abdomen to hold it and the internal organs; the muscles have to do it all. But the abs are just a part of a bigger picture and broader goals that we're going to pursue: strength and flexibility in your entire core region. By that I mean all the muscles in the torso, from your neck to your pubic region—and on both sides, front and back.

To achieve that, we're not just going to work the rectus abdominus, the outermost layer of muscle that runs vertically along your front (that's mostly what sit-ups and crunches will strengthen). To get more multidimensional strength, we'll also work the external obliques that run downward and inward from the ribs, and their counterparts, the internal obliques (they run perpendicular to the externals), which aid in rotation and twisting motions—think golf swing. Yoga exercises also involve the transversus, the deepest (horizontal) layer of ab muscle, which, among other things, aids the expansion and contraction needed in breathing.

Abdominal muscles hold the pelvis and the lower spine in place. Core strength is what allows you to maintain good overall posture, holding the weight of your upper body up so you don't slump down and forward like an old man (no offense to any of our more senior brothers). As Michael, our yoga guru, likes to say, the muscles in this area are "the unsung heroes of the human body."

Even as it promotes stability, the core is literally the center of all motion. The muscles of the abdomen, back and the tops of the glutes are the source from which practically all movement originates—and much of the force with which we do it. Core strength and stability also allow you to maintain balance and control during those movements. From there it's obvious that, in sports, core strength and flexibility are huge keys to superior performance.

Both Eastern and Western schools of thought confirm the importance of the center. In the yoga tradition (and the Indian system of Ayurvedic health), there's a "chakra," or an energy center, right around the solar plexus. Sounds a little dubious to some, but Western medicine makes it seem a lot more plausible. We know, for example, that there are so many nerves in your gut region that some doctors have called it "the second brain." Luckily for us when confronting, say, too much pizza, the other, upstairs brain is really in charge; the lower one is more of a networking and energy distribution hub.

More good news: You're already working the core if you're doing the yoga we've covered so far. For example, in doing that **Killer Yoga Pushup,** you've gotta keep a strong abdomen or you'll collapse downward to the floor. The spinal twists stretch and strengthen the core muscles as well. Here we'll introduce some new yoga moves that have especially good effects on the abs, back and the sides of the torso.

How big of an impact can yoga have on your core? "Huge," says **Diamond Dallas Page,** the former WWE wrestler. "My core strengths in my stomach and my sides and obliques that I've developed are unbelievable." Now that he's got a strong yoga practice going, Dallas reports, "I don't do crunches or sit-ups or any of that crap. They're like a waste of time compared to what I do, and the yoga is way harder than some ab workout. You don't need it; just do the yoga."

THE TRIANGLE

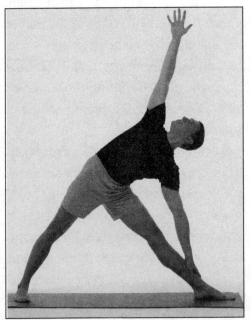

The **Triangle** is one of the great fundamental poses. It's a terrific stretch and strengthener for the legs and the groin, and extends the spine. But I also really like what it does for the core. This sideways lean really lengthens your sides, from the hips all the way up through your neck. To a lesser extent, it also opens the front of the upper torso. The **Triangle** is very complex, so learning to do this one properly will take some patience. Got any?

◆ Stand with your feet about 4 feet apart, a little more if you're over 6 feet. Extend your arms out to the sides, palms facing the mat.

◆ Turn your left foot outward, so your toes are pointing as directly sideways as you can get them. Your knee should be pointing the same way, but your head and torso are still facing front. Now turn the right toes inward a little, to your left. Your left heel should be in line with your right arch. Thigh muscles are engaged, firm.

◆ Inhale and cock your right hip out to the side, away from the center of your body. This will make it easier when you now a) begin exhaling and b) start reaching out to the left with your left hand and extending your torso in that direction. It really helps here to reach *out*—think sideways, not down—and keep extending to the left as far as you can. Dig in with your right heel to anchor yourself.

◆ When you've stretched as far as you can to the left, you're ready to go downward and form the triangle for which this pose is named. Lower the left arm and take hold of your shin below the left knee, resting some of your weight there as you lift the right arm—both are still straight—and raise it up in the air, right hand pointing toward the ceiling. Both arms form one line, at roughly the level of your shoulders. You should feel a nice stretch in the right side of your trunk.

◆ Turn your head and look up at your right fingertips. Note: If you have neck problems, just keep facing front. Stay this way for 5 full breaths at first, then inhale and carefully raise the torso back upward, turning the toes front and breaking the pose.

◆ Rest and repeat on other side. Remember to turn the right toes out fully (and left toes in slightly) as you begin.

As you get stronger and more flexible, you will be able to lower the lead arm further, so that you can rest it lower on the shin, on the ankle and eventually rest it on the ground just in front of your foot. But for now, try to keep your form and angles correct more than worrying about how low you get.

Remember, even though it may seem like all the action is in the front leg, the back one shouldn't just be along for the ride.

Concentrate on keeping it active and involved. "Muscle energy!"

The **Half Boat** and its tougher cousin, the **Full Boat,** work the front abs or rectus abdominus as well as the hip flexors, the stabilizers that run between the inner thighs and the front of the spine.

HALF BOAT

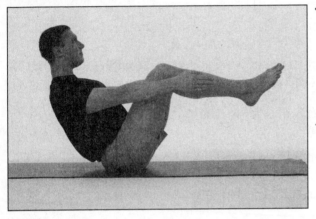

◆ Sit on the mat with your knees up. Arms are down by your sides.

◆ Extend your arms out in front of you, palms facing each other. Inhale and balance there, with your weight on both "sit bones" on either side of your upper butt, rather than the single balance point of your tailbone.

◆ Exhale and lift both legs, keeping them bent at the knees, the insides of your feet touching. Calves are basically parallel to the ground. Your arms are extended on either side of your legs. Use your ab strength to keep your back straight—don't cave in or slump down—and balanced on the narrow perch of your sit bones.

◆ Stay balanced and straight for 5 to 10 full breaths, as long as you can. Keep the oxygen flowing! As always, you want to keep the seemingly secondary body parts active: Really reach out with the arms and tighten them some, so you can feel the biceps and forearms fire.

◆ On an exhale, lower your feet and arms.

◆ Repeat twice more.

SUPER-CHARGE IT!

In the **Full Boat,** you do everything the same way except you straighten the legs. Again, keep them together with the feet touching. You're basically trying to hold your lower and upper halves at right angles to each other. To do that, the core muscles really have to answer the call. If you can't do this without curving the back, go back to the **Half Boat.**

The **Locust** poses put more emphasis on the back of your core. It strengthens the erector spinae muscles, which run on both sides of the spine from the pelvis to the upper back. Like it sounds, this erector set supports the spine and allows us to bend backward through their contraction. Why is this called the **Locust**? You got me—anyone know what a locust looks like? As for a **Half Locust,** I don't even want to think about what that would look like.

HALF LOCUST

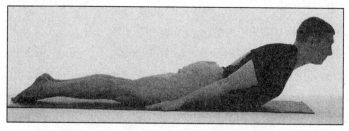

◆ Lie face down on the mat with your arms down by your sides.

◆ Inhale and lift your head and upper chest off the mat. Only lift a few inches; that should be enough to have everything above your breastbone up in the air. Amazing how much your head and that small portion of your body weigh, isn't it?

◆ Try to keep your gaze downward at the mat rather than arching your neck backward; you don't want to hyperextend.

◆ Hold for 5 full breaths, then lower your head and chest back to the mat.

◆ Rest and repeat 3 times.

FULL LOCUST

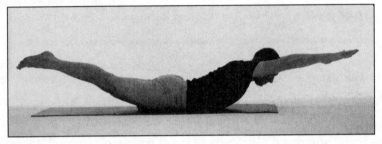

◆ Begin the same way, lying face down, but this time have your arms fully extended out in front of you.

◆ Inhale, and as you raise your upper torso, lift up your arms as well, either thumbs up or palms down (as shown here). This makes the weight you're holding up with your back and ab muscles greater by two arms' worth.

◆ To increase the difficulty even more: Raise your legs off the ground as well, so your entire body is balanced on your abdomen and pelvis area. This brings the lower back muscles strongly into play. Remember to look down, not up, and breathe fully in and out. All in all, it's one tough locust.

Mini-Workout Update: You can now add in some of the strength, balance, breathing or core exercises to the 10 flexibility moves we did earlier. You pick 'em, but for now, stay away from the Super-Charged variations. I'd also lay off the **Wheel** and stick to the **Pigeon Variation**, not the killer **Pigeon**.

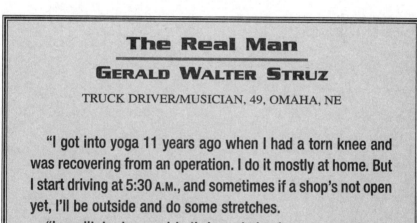

The Real Man

GERALD WALTER STRUZ

TRUCK DRIVER/MUSICIAN, 49, OMAHA, NE

"I got into yoga 11 years ago when I had a torn knee and was recovering from an operation. I do it mostly at home. But I start driving at 5:30 A.M., and sometimes if a shop's not open yet, I'll be outside and do some stretches.

"I meditate, too, and both have helped me tremendously dealing with the stress of my job. I don't honk and get road rage in the cab. They've also helped my focus in playing guitar at a coffee shop here. I play there every month or so and it makes me more calm. I don't get nervous when tons of people come and boo me or cheer.

"If you tell people that I practice yoga and have a truck-driving job—they're like, 'Yoga, isn't that for women?' I say, 'In India it's mostly men that do it.' I just say it's been good for me and point out a few reasons why, and I always point out that it's not for everybody. But I've recommended it to just about everybody I know."

CHAPTER 9

Injuries: Prevention & Recovery

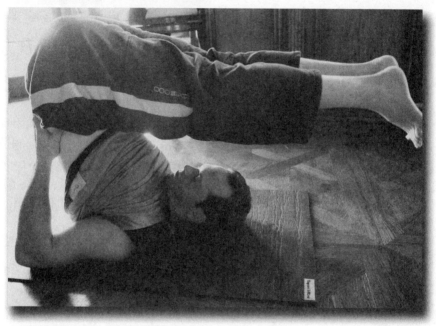

All-Star catcher Mike Lieberthal in the Plough. "I took up yoga for flexibility, but it's important for injury rehab, too. After surgery, it helped me get the flexibility and strength back in my knee."

How's this for Real Men doing yoga? In El Monte, California, there's a firehouse run by Captain Bob Hagg. Hagg, 47, is also the leader of a Special Operations unit in an anti-terrorist task force. He's 6'3", 230 pounds—and he's had his firehouse doing yoga for "two or three years now." Why?

"It lessens the injuries," says Captain Hagg. "We get in awkward positions: crawling inside a smashed-up vehicle, or swinging an ax and dragging a hose upstairs, things like that. That's where a lot of guys were getting hurt, but we haven't had that since we started doing yoga. Also, after a fire it would take a couple of days to recover, and it doesn't take as hard a toll on our bodies when we practice.

"We all do it together for an hour. We put in a videotape and follow that. We use Rodney Yee. We have yoga mats and blocks and straps for some of us. We do cardio and weights, but the thing is, yoga gives you more flexibility. At the end of the exercise, we take time to meditate. We've gone to different studios together, too, on days off, and it builds camaraderie as well."

Just like athletes, lots of other tough guys—or guys who are tough on their bodies—are taking to the mat to prevent injuries. The main principle's the same for all: Greater flexibility means greater chances of staying healthy. Baseball yoga guru Alan Jaeger puts it in terms of his sport, but ones we can all relate to. "When you can train the muscle through a deeper, longer stretch, it responds more positively," he says. "It's got more strength and can take more punishment. That way, in the eighth inning of a game when someone else might begin tightening up, your muscles have greater endurance and you'll be in less of a position to get hurt."

Keith Washington, a 275-pound defensive end for the Denver Broncos does yoga for an hour and a half every Friday during the season with instructor Danny Poole. He took some persuading from some of his teammates before he tried it. "That's because I didn't know much about it," he says. "I'm thinking 'Yoga—you hum and you chant.'" But now he's a believer, and injury prevention is his primary goal. "You stretch your muscles to the extreme," he says, "to the point that it's almost painful, then you breathe and relax. So now if I were to go out and get an ankle sprain, let's say, my muscles won't be shocked because they've stretched, stressed to that point. It's like, 'Okay, we've been here before.' That's huge."

It's not just how far you stretch, Washington knows, it's also how long you hold that stretch. "You get in a position and hold it for a minute or so as opposed to on the football field where you'll just go down [in an awkward position] for a few seconds. So you're actually shocking your muscles beyond the time that you might go."

The Real Man

DAVE HERNDON

JOURNALIST, 46, NEW YORK CITY

Author's note: Dave is a good friend of mine, the guy who introduced me to yoga. He first took up yoga after he blew out a knee—doing windsprints with me, I'm afraid. He had a knee operation, and he's had to give up the high-impact sports. However, yoga's helped him to be Joe Active again. Here, I'll let him tell it:

"I've got nasty arthritis in that knee, and squash was killing me—the knee swelled like a grapefruit. My orthopedist said I was cruising straight for knee replacement and he prescribed some tedious strengthening exercises, which I promptly abandoned. Instead, I do yoga now, and get a total body workout that's enjoyable and easy on the knees (I do avoid some of the kneeling postures). Now when I go snowboarding, I do a little yoga warm-up before I start, and instead of being an arthritic gimp out there, I feel like I've still got some juice in those 40-something legs."

Since signing as a free-agent for the 1997 season, Washington has not missed a game due to injury. "Even when we're on the field on game day I sometimes apply some of the stretches," he reports. "I'm hoping to enable myself to go a little longer in this game."

What's the best way to prevent the Big Hurt? As you no doubt know already, it's important to warm up properly, to get the muscles warm and your joints loose, before any strenuous activity. Most trainers recommend a short cardio interval, followed by stretching, before beginning the run or lifting or what-have-you. Let's face it, though: Who has time—or the patience—for a two-stage, not-very-interesting warm-up period before we can get going? If your life and schedule are anything like mine, that takes too long.

Plus, the stretching part has recently been called into question in a major way. A recent study of traditional, static stretching done in Australia sent shock waves through the fitness community. It followed more than twenty-five hundred recruits in the Aussie army, some of whom stretched before training and some of whom didn't. The researchers concluded that static stretching did nothing to prevent injuries. That's zippo, nada, zilch. So the army dropped it from its routine. "We're not suggesting that people not warm up," said the physiology professor who supervised the experiments. "The only thing that's a waste of time is this form of static stretching before exercise."

What's a jocky guy to do? What you need to warm up is "dynamic stretching," a flowing series of stretches in which each is held briefly, then you move fairly quickly to the next. This brisk movement sequence allows you to stretch many more muscle groups in the same amount of time and also has the advantage of getting your heart rate up, so you're combining the two stages of the traditional warm-up— cardio and stretching—into one much more efficient period.

At this point you won't be surprised to hear that there's a yoga practice that fits this bill. It's called the **Sun Salute,** as it was traditionally done in the morning to wake the body up and start the day. We'll be using it as a warm-up early on in our rookies and veterans routines.

The **Sun Salute** incorporates many yoga postures that we've already learned, so it's another opportunity to hone your technique. Basically, we'll be moving to the rhythm of the breath, one move on the inhale, and the next on the exhale, so doing this will also get you focused on your breathing.

After you've used this sequence to warm up for yoga, you can start using it as a warm-up for your other sports activities. And on days when you don't have time for much exercise of any kind, just a couple rounds can keep you from locking up between workouts.

SUN SALUTE

◆ Stand on your mat, feet about hip width apart, hands down or in prayer position at the center of your chest.

◆ Inhale slowly, raising your arms overhead, and gently arch backward. You can leave your hands in prayer, hook the thumbs together, or let the arms come apart. Before you begin to bend backward, think about stretching and extending up first, lengthening to your highest extent, before beginning the arch. Only bend as far as feels comfortable and safe; you can go farther when you get more warmed up.

◆ On the next exhale, come back to vertical and then continue forward, leading with your arms and hands, bending at the hips and folding your upper body downward to meet your legs in the **Standing Forward Bend** (this is great for the back; see the next chapter). Place your hands on the ground on either side of your feet. Bend your knees if you need to accomplish that and to assure there's very little space between your thighs and your chest. Your head is down, facing the wall behind you.

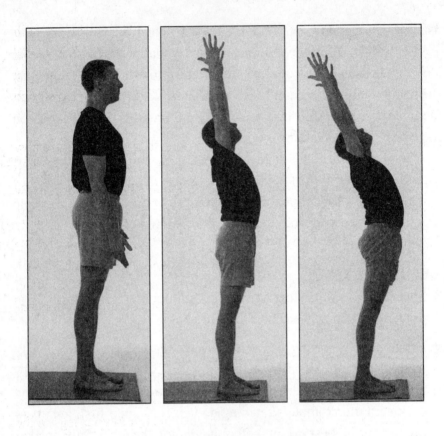

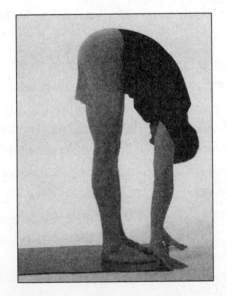

◆ Inhale and extend the right leg back behind you in a lunge, with your left leg bent, left foot flat on the ground between your hands. Raise up your head and torso so you're looking at the ceiling or a high part of the wall in front of you. This will help you put a stretch into your inner thighs.

◆ Exhale and extend the left leg back to meet the right, so you're now supporting your body with your extended arms and feet in a pushup position. Keep your body in a straight line—**Plank** position. Now you're giving the arm and shoulder muscles a little warm-up.

◆ Segue right into the **Cobra** pose we've already learned by lowering your knees to the mat, then your chest, then your forehead. Your arms are still bent on either side of you in pre-pushup style. Then, on the inhale, raise your head and torso off the ground, bending from the lower back.

◆ Next, exhale and push your upper body up off the floor with your arms as you bring your chest and head forward and down out of the **Cobra.** Keep lowering your straightened-out torso down toward the floor as you raise your hips and push back into your legs in the **Downward Dog.**

◆ Inhale and step the right foot underneath you and forward, into the lunge you were in before, except this time your right leg is bent, the left leg still extended behind you. Raise your chest up and look up again.

◆ Exhale and bring the left foot forward to meet the right, folding forward over your legs again in the **Standing Forward Bend.**

◆ Inhale and unfold your body, elevating your head and torso back toward vertical. Prolong the inhale and keep going into the backward bend we did at the very beginning of the sequence. As before, stretch your arms fully upward before arching backward.

◆ Exhale and come back to the upright standing position and return

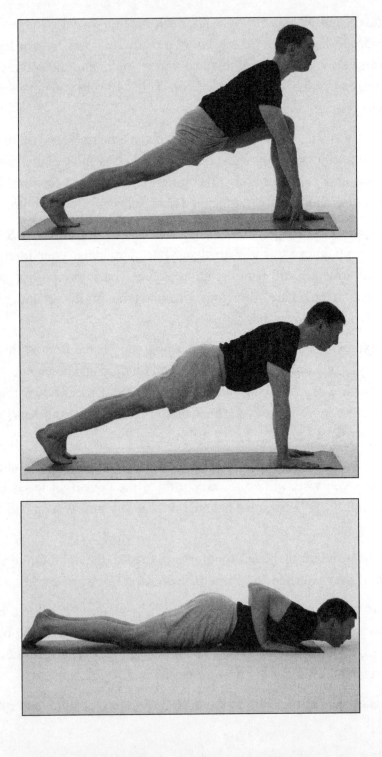

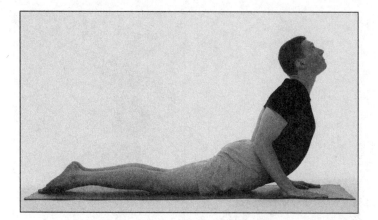

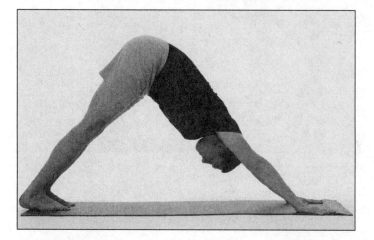

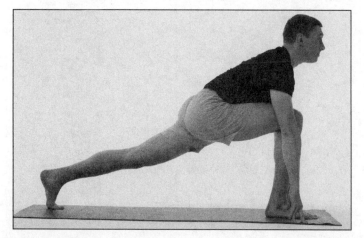

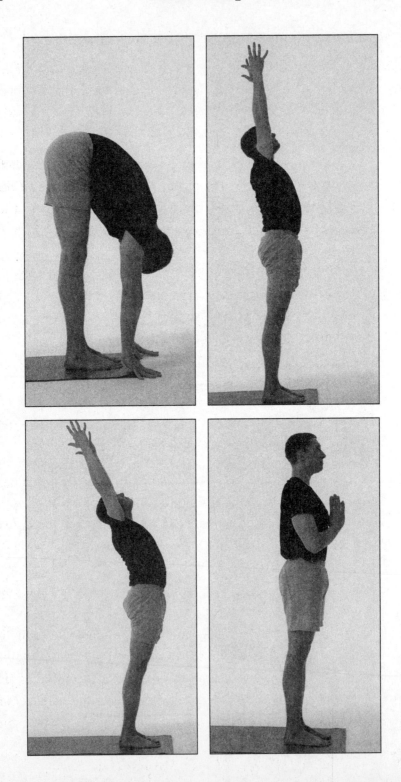

the hands to prayer in the center of your chest. That's 1 rep.

◆ Repeat the entire sequence, but this time start by kicking the left leg back from the forward bend, so you reverse the stretches. Concentrate on breathing fully and keeping your movements in synch with your inhales and exhales.

After that, you should feel warmed and loose all over, maybe huffing and puffing a little bit—in other words, ready to go! A full **Sun Salute** consists of one sequence that starts by kicking the right leg back and another round that starts with moving the left leg back.

Mini-Workout Update: Start adding two or three of these to your ongoing exercise sessions. Do them first thing, before your upper-body stretches.

RECOVERING FROM INJURIES

No matter how good your precautions, injuries are still gonna happen. And when they do, yoga will still be there for you. First, your injuries may be less severe if you've been practicing. "Maybe instead of missing two or three games," says Denver's Danny Poole, "a player will miss just one; the trauma won't be as severe." As more and more doctors and physical therapists are coming around to believing, yoga will help you to recover better and faster.

That's what Phillies catcher **Mike Lieberthal** found out during the 2001 season, when he was diving back to first on a pick-off attempt and tore the ACL, MCL and lateral meniscus in his right knee. He missed the rest of the season, had surgery to repair the damage and incorporated yoga into his rehabilitation. "I took up yoga in the first place for flexibility; that's so important for a catcher," he says. "But I found out it's important for rehabilitation, too. You need to get your flexibility and strength back after surgery. You do a lot of balancing on one leg holding the poses, and that helps with the flexibility, strength and stability in the knee."

Opening up the joints and improving blood flow to the injured area hastens recovery. The same healing process helps you cope with overuse, and wear and tear that's rough on your body but stops short of an out-and-out injury.

In the NBA, for example, it's not just the games; it's so many games in so few nights, plus the travel, that wears players down. Troy Wenzel, athletic trainer of the Milwaukee Bucks, has brought in yoga instructors to try to combat this fatigue/injury syndrome. "I see clear benefit," Wenzel says. "The breathing techniques get more oxygen into the system, promoting healing and recovery, more red blood cells . . . plus there's stress reduction, relaxation and flexibility benefits, so it's really like three or five things in one."

Injury prevention plus better recuperation through yoga allow you to keep practicing the sports and activities that you love. However, there is such a thing as:

YOGA INJURIES

Yep, they happen. Yoga advocates don't like to talk about it, but people hurt themselves all the time. The two biggest reasons are beginners trying to do more than they're capable of, and yoga instructors who don't know what they're doing. Sometimes, of course, those two risk factors are combined.

With yoga exploding in popularity, doctors and physical therapists say they're seeing more muscle and cartilage tears, ligament sprains and disk injuries. A recent *Boston Globe* article compared this upsurge to the injuries that happened when high-impact aerobics took off in the 1980s.

Hey, from what you've done so far, you know yoga is no joke. So don't be an idiot. Or, to be a little nicer about it, don't try to be a yoga superhero. Get into the stretches as deeply as your body allows, then very gently try to extend your capabilities. No kamikaze lunges or grabs for glory. Again: It doesn't matter what the guy or girl next to you in class is doing—or, for that matter, what the model in this book's pictures is doing. Do what you can do. And if something starts to hurt, stop doing it. Remember, we're in this for the long haul.

As far as teachers and classes go, be leery of anyone who takes a super-gung-ho, go-for-broke approach. Yoga shouldn't hurt, and anyone who encourages you to fight through the pain is off-base. A good teacher will offer options at various points in a class, describing different ways that the inexperienced and the experienced can approach a certain pose. In Michael's classes, he calls that Level One and Level Two. Ask what training a yoga teacher's had; "affiliation" is good, "certified" is usually better. Generally speaking, teachers trained in the Iyengar and Anusara traditions are good to start with because of their emphasis on alignment. Unfortunately, though, many teachers out there are clueless—proceed with caution.

One thing to watch out for: Instructors will sometimes come around and "help" the inflexible by giving them a gentle—or not so gentle—push to deepen their stretches. Until you are sure they have the knowledge and judgment to do that properly, just tell them nicely to back off. I mean it: I don't let anyone I don't know push me into stretches. I'm polite about it, but firm. It's my back, Jack.

Remember, too, though, that yoga is essentially safe. These positions have been used for five thousand years and if they habitually injured folks, there wouldn't *be* any yoga. In that same *Boston Globe* article about injuries, Jack Kennedy of the Massachusetts Governor's Committee on Physical Fitness and Sports says that: "In general, yoga is safer than most types of exercise. . . . But when you have something trendy, you have people trying to take it to the limit." Just don't be one of these trendy extremists, and you'll be fine.

Yoga Jocks

Amani Toomer

WIDE RECEIVER, NEW YORK GIANTS

"My wife started me off on it. She took me to my first yoga class out in California several years ago. Then I started doing it in the off-season. It was hard but a great workout. It helps me with flexibility—you get a lot of motion in your body that you wouldn't normally get. So I feel like I can move a little bit better, and the better you can move, the quicker you can be and the less likely you are to get injured.

"Yoga also really helped me with my balance, my abdominal strength and overall strength. It's the strength that you get from holding a pose. Not weight-lifting strength, but real functional body strength.

"Every player on this team who's done it definitely respects it. And I would definitely recommend it to anyone. In fact, I have a brother who just tore his Achilles tendon, and I told him, 'You should have been doing yoga.'

"I'll be doing yoga long after I stop playing football. I won't lift weights or anything like that. I'll do yoga.'"

CHAPTER 10
No More Back Pain!

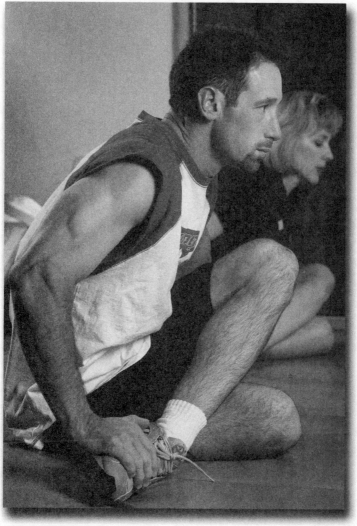

©Paul F. Gero, 2003

Arizona Diamondbacks slugger Luis Gonzales uses yoga moves to de-stress, stretch and strengthen his lower back.

Yoga saved my career."

That's **Justin Gimelstob,** 26, professional tennis player. At this writing he's won nine doubles titles and two mixed doubles titles (with Venus Williams). In singles, he's made it to the third round of the U.S. Open and Wimbledon.

But three years ago he was going nowhere. "I had back problems, two herniated disks," he remembers. "Everything was locked up, and the pain was so bad I could barely move around on the court. I had nine cortisone shots, and I was taking tremendous amounts of Vicodin.

"I was looking at surgery; my doctors wanted me to have it. I thought I would definitely lose range of motion and there'd be a long rehab and, you know, the results are never guaranteed. . . . It was a very emotional time for me. You're 23 or 24 and looking at your career possibly being over.

"I was going to do it. I remember meeting with my dad in a hotel room one night to decide. I started crying; we were both really sad. But then Alex O'Brian, my doubles partner, said, 'Before you do that, you should try yoga.'"

Gimelstob hired Los Angeles instructor Jennifer Greenhut, and she traveled with him for a while on the tour. "It just took a couple weeks for me to see a difference," he says. "I haven't taken a pill since. I haven't had back pain since. It's been unbelievable."

Now he takes classes at least three times a week. "Initially the benefits were centered around my back problem," says the 6'5", 190-pound Gimelstob. "But after that, the most important poses for me have been for my hips. It helps me after a long day of practice; it opens up my hips, shoulders and groin. In tennis, my movement and balance are better, and my muscles are more relaxed now, less rigid. Plus, getting in touch with my breathing has also helped me as far as staying calm and in control. I had a tendency to get wound up and go faster and faster; now in a match I'll focus on my breathing and my diaphragm, things we work on in classes, and it'll calm me down.

"I rave about yoga," Gimelstob concludes. "I'm a total convert."

More than 6 million Americans suffer from lower back pain (the most common kind) each year. Over 80 percent will experience some back problem in their lifetimes. Most back pain is acute and will resolve itself within three weeks, but anyone with a chronically bad back will tell you that it can cast misery over your entire life. That's because so much of what we do—basically, everything—involves that finicky spinal column.

You may have even heard the notion that man wasn't originally designed to walk upright, and that carrying our weight this way is why we have so many back problems. There could be some truth to it; one of the biggest problems with backs is compression. In fact, humans are born with 33 vertebrae and over time those fuse into just 24. But what are you going to do—the walking upright thing is probably here to stay, don't you think?

As with flexibility problems, back pain is rooted in both activity and inactivity. We know that sedentary lifestyles and poor posture play major roles. For Boomers, age also plays a part. Bone density is gradually lost—by men, as well as women—and our ligaments and tendons shorten as we age, so range of motion is diminished. Recreational sports, falls, car accidents and the like can all rack up the back. One example of men whose back pain has a traumatic onset, points out Danny Poole, is football linemen. "All they do is crash into the other team, over and over," he says, "so the vertebrae get compressed."

For guys with less violent lifestyles, garden-variety hamstring tightness is an extremely common problem, says Jennifer Greenhut, Gimelstob's yoga teacher. "When they get tight, the pelvis is pulled forward and rotated improperly and the lower back is put into sway. That's what happened with Justin: His spine was compressed."

So the question becomes: What can we do about our aching backs?

Many people find that drugs, both painkillers and anti-inflammatories, provide only temporary relief because the pain is based in an ongoing mechanical problem. Surgeries, as Gimelstob points out, are drastic measures with uncertain results. Some people swear by chiropractic, but not all.

More active people often try to work their way out of back trouble. In recent years, the conventional wisdom has been: "You need to work the abs, because they support the lower back." And countless sufferers are busily crunching away. But new evidence suggests that ab work is far from a magic bullet. *Yoga Journal* recently reported on a fascinating study in which male and female college athletes who used traditional core-strengthening exercises were just as likely to develop back pain as those who did not.

Increasingly, a gentle approach to yoga is becoming the therapy of first resort for back-pain sufferers—and more doctors as well. It's non-invasive, nontraumatic, no drugs needed. Those factors alone make it worth a try—but in researching this book I also heard from a jillion guys (give or take) that for them, yoga was a genuine back-saver.

Jonathan Kelley, who runs a pizza restaurant in Mentor, Ohio, started having back problems a couple of years ago. "At my job, I'm on my feet a lot," says the 32-year-old. "Plus, I pulled a muscle. So I was working with a masseuse and that fixed the problems temporarily, but then I'd keep re-injuring myself. It was expensive, too. In the spring of 2000, I tried yoga. My back felt better almost instantly. Now I don't go to the masseuse. I don't need it. And my posture is much better since I started yoga. On my job I'm able to stand straight up and work better."

Since yoga treats the total body, it can also help alleviate problems that are felt in the back, but don't necessarily originate right there. Often, says New York trainer and flexibility expert Paul Frediani, "If you stretch out the shoulders and the hip flexors, the lower back will take care of itself." Many other experts believe that back problems can be psychological or rooted in stress, which yoga helps relieve, too (more on that later).

Please note that if you suffer from persistent back pain that's at all severe, you should consult with doctors before you self-treat with yoga or anything else—you could make the problem worse.

That being said, many of the poses we've already learned

will support and relieve the back. They include:

Crescent Moon, the **Warrior** series and the **Triangle**—really good for the hip flexors and psoas.

Downward Dog, Hamstring Stretch and the **Forward Bends**—they loosen the hamstrings, which, says Jennifer Greenhut, "allows the pelvis to lower back to its proper position."

Pigeon—as we noted earlier, it stretches out the piriformus muscle, great for folks with sciatica.

Cobra and the **Spinal Twists**—the backbend and twisting motion help unlock rigid areas. Eric Paskel, who offers classes specifically for back pain at his studio, Sanga Yoga, in the Detroit area, says the twists also "wring out and lubricate the spine, so you flush out old spinal fluid and bring in fresh fluid."

To focus on back relief, you can begin to emphasize these poses more in your yoga workouts, either by adding repetitions of the most therapeutic poses, holding them for longer, or both. Here are three more moves to add into the mix that are also terrific for the lower back.

STANDING FORWARD BEND

We did this fairly quickly in the **Sun Salutes;** here we'll linger longer to prolong the stretch. You'll be using gravity and the weight of your torso to gently lengthen out your hamstrings, lower back, hips, calves and Achilles.

With the leg muscles properly firing and engaged, this bend (or forward fold) is also a strengthener for the quads and calf muscles. Using gravity as your guide, this position can also be a great way to mark your progress over time. See how far you are able to extend down toward the floor at the beginning, and you'll be really pleased to see your reach gradually improve.

But not yet. Don't try to be a Yoga Achiever here or start competing with yourself to get farther down in this bend. We're dealing with your vulnerable lower back. This pose can be extremely beneficial, but it's absolutely vital that you do not force or overdo.

To help you ease into it, do this exercise with the knees bent for the first 2 to 3 weeks and see how it goes. Everyone—whether you think you have a really tight lower back or not. Then try to straighten your legs slowly and gradually, as taught below.

If you've got back problems, place a chair at arms-length in front of you and when you fold forward, place your hands on the top, the arms or the seat of the chair instead of reaching down further toward the floor. Just bend as far as you can comfortably go and feel a stretch at the same time. You can also try resting your forearms on the chair for support.

The standard version goes like this:

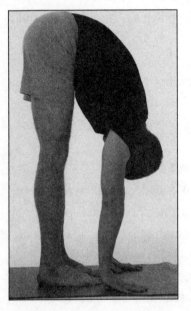

◆ Stand on your mat. Inhale and extend your arms fully overhead (without raising the shoulder blades).

◆ Exhale strongly, and as you do, reach forward and outward, toward the facing wall, shifting your weight that way. Remember, this is a *forward* bend; the stretch in this direction will help you to get farther in the next direction (downward). Think of lengthening the front torso first, then lowering it.

◆ Continuing the same motion, bend at the hips—not the waist—and then begin reaching your hands and arms down toward the floor instead of forward. As they descend, they gently pull the head and torso, which follow along behind.

◆ Have your knees straight if possible (see above), but it's more important that they not be locked. When you're at reach the end of your reach, just let the hands, arms and upper body hang over your legs wherever they've stopped.

◆ Make sure your feet are feel well-grounded into the floor, with your weight slightly forward or evenly distributed on the soles. Don't lean backward.

◆ Your leg muscles, especially in the front of the thighs, should be working hard. Keep them active.

◆ Don't force yourself to descend any farther, and don't try to extend your head and neck to reach downward. Head and neck are loose, dangling.

◆ Breathe strongly and fully, in and out. See if you feel yourself extending downward very slightly on the exhales. After you've done this pose for a while, you can try more consciously to make that happen. But while you're new to it, just hang—and breathe. Stay there for 10 full breaths. (As you progress, work up to 15 breaths, then a full minute.)

◆ On an inhale, break the pose by extending the arms back out in front of you, lengthening the front torso again.

◆ Continue to straighten, lifting your head and trunk and reaching the arms overhead as in the first phase of the pose. Come all the way back to standing.

If you feel sharp pain anywhere during this exercise, stop immediately.

SEATED FORWARD BEND

The Sanskrit name for this variation is *Paschimottanasana,* which translates as "intense stretch of the west." But it's actually less intense than the standing version. Consider it as a substitute for the **Standing Forward Bend** if you have a touchy back; otherwise, add it in as a supplemental back exercise.

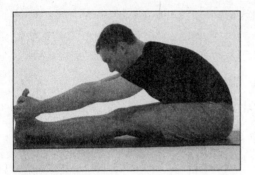

◆ Sit on the mat with your legs extended out in front of you, heels close together.

◆ Inhale, and raise both arms high overhead, stretching upward through the hands and fingers.

◆ Exhale and fold forward from the hips, reaching your extended arms out and down toward your feet. Try to reach outward or forward, keeping your upper body long rather than slumping downward toward your thighs.

◆ Ideally, you grab the sides of the feet with your hands. If not, just reach out as far as you can comfortably go and let the hands fall where they may. Or, use a strap looped around the soles of your feet to help you into the stretch.

◆ Hold for 10 full breaths (optional: work up to 1 minute). On the exhales, try to extend a little bit more—gently—then relax back a bit on the inhales.

◆ Inhale and return to sitting.

Since this is lower impact than the standing pose, you can probably hold it longer without strain. For a real back therapy session, shoot for 5 minutes.

THE BRIDGE

This works the legs very vigorously, but also stretches the neck and spine—and it really made my lower back feel better. Hope it works for you, too.

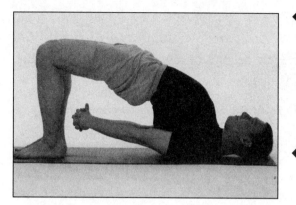

◆ Lie on your back with your knees bent and your feet on the mat, heels close to your butt. Arms are down by your side.

◆ Exhale and push off the floor with your legs and feet, raising your hips and rear off the floor. Push up as high as you can without feeling strain in the lower back. Try to get your thighs parallel to the floor. Your weight is now on your heels, the top of your shoulders (where they meet the bottom of your neck) and the back of your head.

◆ To get higher up, you can push with the backs of your arms as well, or try clasping your hands underneath you. But focus your efforts and your muscle energy on lifting your lower back, hips and groin. In addition to pushing up from below, imagine also that you are raising your top side—abdomen, etc.—from above.

◆ Stay in the pose for 30 seconds, maintaining your breathing. Exhale and come down to the floor. Try to roll your back down slowly, vertebrae by vertebrae, starting with the uppermost part and continuing till your sit bones hit the mat.

SUPER-CHARGE IT!

Squeeze a folded towel, a Styrofoam yoga block (available wherever fine yoga accessories are sold) or a big-city phone book between your thighs as you perform the exercise. This will fire the adductors, which opens up the pelvic floor and allows the tailbone to tuck down and under, which puts a little traction into the lumbar spine.

For a longer exploration of yoga and back problems, including a detailed exercise program, I recommend two books by Loren Fishman, M.D., and Carol Ardman. The first is called *Back Pain* (W. W. Norton, 2000) and the second one (as yet untitled), specifically on yoga and backs, is due out in January 2004.

CHAPTER 11

Yoga for Golf Plus: Sport-by-Sport Workouts

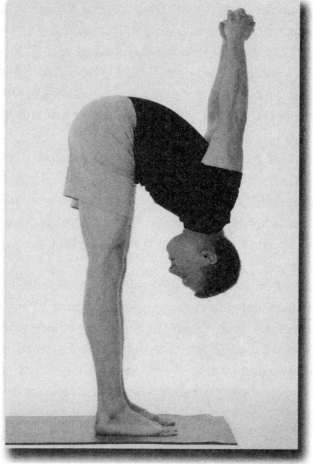

©Erica Berger, 2003

The Arms-Up Forward Bend adds terrific shoulder opening to the version we already learned. And greater range of motion in that joint is key to a more powerful golf swing.

Let's see, what do you need to play your best golf?

Good balance and flexibility, range of motion, functional strength—the exact same qualities that yoga gives you. You also need focus and a strong mental game, and as we'll see in chapter 13, yoga hones that ability to its keenest. The things that yoga doesn't really help you with—cardiovascular endurance and weight-lifter strength—don't matter in golf.

That's why golfers, pro and amateur, have been among the first athletes to embrace yoga. **David Duval,** one of the PGA's best, does 30 minutes of yoga every day; **Jesper Parnevik** practices, too. **Ty Tryon,** the phenom who made the PGA tour at age 17, has his own yoga coach. **Joe Inman,** who plays and is also a color commentator on the Senior Tour, is a major convert (see Yoga Jocks sidebar, this chapter). On the women's side, **Annika Sorenstam** and **Se Ri Pak** do yoga, too.

Not because they want to be one with the universe. They want to be one with that winner's trophy. And they found out that yoga improves your golf from the moment you lift the bag out of the trunk (your greater flexibility preventing a back injury in that awkward motion) to the time you hit the clubhouse, 19th hole or awards ceremony.

Here's a look at the many ways yoga works beautifully for golf, and which poses help you at each stage of the game. Plus, we'll add one new position that seems like it was tailor-made—Taylor Made?—for golf, a variation on the **Standing Forward Bend.** But just by doing yoga regularly, you'll probably take a few strokes off your game—or at the very least, put a potent weapon in your bag.

Warming Up: As Paul Frediani, top trainer and author of *Golf Flex,* points out, "Stretching in the traditional static or passive way does very little to prepare you for the explosive movement of swinging a golf club." The dynamic stretching of yoga, especially the **Sun Salutes** we learned earlier, is a much better preparation, one that gets the entire body ready to go.

The Stance: When you settle in to address the ball, the balance work you've done in yoga—**Tree, Eagle, Warrior III**—helps you ground yourself properly through your legs and feet, feeling a solid connection to the earth. This serves you well when you're teeing off but even more so afterward. Katherine Roberts, a yoga teacher based in Colorado, who's made working with golfers her entire business, points out that "there are tons of stabilizing issues" inherent in the game. "When you're in a bunker, in a bad lie—you really have to play from all angles," she says. "After all, the average golfer probably hits the ball 105 times and you only get to hit the ball from a level, teed-up position 18 times."

Thanks to the strength poses for the legs like **Warrior I** and **II,** the **Bridge** and the **Bow,** you're strong in your stance. All the strengthening of the core muscles, the erector spinae, and the spine itself in poses such as the **Locust, Boat** and **Cobra,** allow you to stand more erect. Your breath work also sets you up to succeed here. Roberts teaches her clients to "incorporate deep, diaphragmatic breathing into their preshot routine. As you take those breaths, envision all tension leaving your body and you will consciously relax all your muscles. Then inhale as you begin your backswing or takeaway. . . ."

The Backswing: Here's where the hip and shoulder openers we've learned—**Pigeon, Half Eagle**—really pay off. The greater flexibility you've gained in those joints means you can rotate more deeply as you coil into your backswing. That improved range of motion extends the length or radius of your swing, and that means you can strike through with greater power.

PGA golfer **J. L. Lewis** finished in the top 10 at four tournaments last year, earning just under a million dollars. He took up yoga in 1997. "Flexibility is the most important thing for a golfer," he says. "All the stretches made my swing longer—there's no question about it. I got back farther while maintaining my balance. The added range of motion enabled me to get a better turn and power through the ball. The **Downward Dog, Standing Forward Bend** and others helped stretch out my back, hips and shoulders. And holding those positions while I breathed really helped keep my body loose."

Yoga poses that develop the obliques, such as the **Triangle,** give you even more power in the backswing. On her Web site, *yoga forgolfers.com,* Katherine Roberts cites medical evidence that "Ninety-five percent of the muscular effort involved in creating torso rotation comes from your oblique abdominal muscles."

The Swing: As you exhale and bring the club forward, the hip openers will help you access the muscles in your glutes, among the biggest and strongest in the body. As Sarah Pryor, yoga coach to young PGA-er Ty Tryon says, "On most men, the hip flexors are like concrete." As we've discussed, the psoas and piriformus muscles are also locked tight on many guys. But not yours—you do yoga! **Pigeon's** a favorite of Tryon, Pryor says, also citing **Triangle** and the **Warrior** poses for improving lower body flexibility. Throughout the swing, you're maintaining your balance as you shift your weight, just as you've done so many times on the mat.

The Follow Through: Here's the second stage at which your increased range of motion in the hips and shoulder lengthens the arc of the swing, generating more power. When you're finishing, you want to rotate your torso so far around that your belt buckle ends up pointing at the target, in line with the hole. "Many people don't have that kind of rotation," says Sarah Pryor. "But golfers who do yoga can get it." Thank the **Kneeling Twist** and **Seated Twist.**

Injury Prevention: Just as in other sports, yoga keeps you in the game. Golf may not seem like the most violent or dangerous pursuit, but over time the golf swing puts a lot of wear and tear on the body and injuries are frequent. You're using something like 70 muscles to explode into your swing from a static position and you're doing it around 100 times an outing (if it's less, congrats to you). Opening and strengthening the arms and upper body in yoga helps prevent elbow tendonitis and shoulder injuries, especially in the rotator cuffs. Hamstring flexibility wards off lower-back strain—extremely common among golfers—and supports the knee flexion you need on the course. And the twists support the constant coiling and uncoiling in the swing, the kind of repetitive motion that can otherwise lead to overuse injuries.

Part of the injury risk in golf is the asymmetry inherent in all one-sided games. Because you always swing from one side, your muscles will be more developed on the dominant side. These stronger muscles tend to be tighter, which limits range of motion, while the weaker muscles tend to be more flexible. Your regular yoga routine will work both sides equally, which helps, but to create more symmetry prominent yoga teacher Baron Baptiste recommends that golfers add a little extra work. Hold strengthening poses like the **Side Plank** longer on the weaker side of your body to compensate for that imbalance. To give an extra stretch to the bigger, tighter muscles, hold lengthening poses—including **Triangle**—longer on your stronger, dominant side.

The Mental Game: It was the night before the last round of Q-School in 2001; the next day's play would determine who would qualify for the PGA Pro Tour the next year. Ty Tryon sat meditating on the California golf course that night with his yoga teacher, using breathing techniques to instill deep relaxation. Tryon sat motionless, visualizing himself playing at his highest potential. Then he rose and announced, "I'm gonna shoot a 65 and pull this off." The next day he shot a 6-under-par 66, and became the youngest person to ever qualify for the PGA tour—at age 17.

Pryor, a certified Bikram and Ashtanga instructor, has worked with him for two years or more now (she works with pro tennis players as well). For her, yoga's mental benefits for golf begin with the breath. "It's one of the few things in the body we can really control," she says. "And doing that allows you to calm yourself on the back nine."

Pryor also teaches that yoga discipline instills mental toughness that pays off on the golf course. "Some of the poses are uncomfortable and you want to come right out of them," she says. "But the pose really begins at that instant when you want to come out of it, and you just have to hang in there. It's the same as in the athlete's profession: You can't just stop the game and walk away when you feel like it."

There you have 'em: a whole bag full of physical and mental tools that will improve your golf game. As Katherine Roberts asks: "What piece of titanium is going to give you all that?"

On top of all that, here's another pose that could have been created specifically with golfers in mind. (No word on this in the yoga sutras, or original texts, but who knows? Maybe they just forgot to mention golf.) In this variation on the **Standing Forward Bend,** you are not only working the legs—and waking up the hamstrings, calves and quads pre–tee-off—but the arm action *really* loosens up the upper body in ways that facilitate the golf swing. Your shoulder joints and blades get limber, as do the lower back and neck. Plus, pulling the arms overhead opens up the core's intercostal muscles (on the sides, between the ribs), which, as noted, generates a lot of your power. See how our model Glen does this in the photo opening this chapter.

ARMS-UP FORWARD BEND

◆ Stand erect with arms extended behind you, away from the body, and hands clasped.

◆ Breathe in deeply. Then, on the exhale, bend forward from the hips and fold your torso down toward your thighs, lowering your head as low as you can go toward the floor and moving your chest as close as possible to your legs.

◆ As the upper body descends, raise the arms up behind you, keeping them straight and fully extended. Let your head hang loosely, facing your legs.

◆ Don't forget about the legs. Keep them strong and engaged—but the knees are not locked.

◆ Ideally, your clasped hands are now directly over your head. Breathe deeply as you hold this position for 30 seconds. During that time, if your shoulders loosen and you can raise the arms higher, go for it. But don't yank. To get the torso folded over more and the head lower, you can bend your knees. This will in turn cant the arms further forward into the stretch.

◆ Inhale as you come back up, and release the arms.

◆ Repeat twice more. Try to hold for 45 seconds the second time and then for a full minute on the third rep.

SPORT-BY-SPORT

Here's a look at other sports and activities you may enjoy, the physical challenges they present, and the yoga positions that most directly address those needs. You can emphasize these prescriptive or corrective positions in your yoga workouts by adding an extra rep or two. At the least, make sure you are doing them properly and attentively.

Of course, the overall flexibility you gain from yoga will benefit you in all sports. And the breathing exercises will help your stamina and performance across the board. Just being more aware of what you're demanding of your body when you run, roller blade or what-have-you can help prevent injuries. Remember, too, that the **Sun Salute** sequence is a great warm-up *and* cool-down; try doing about 5 minutes' worth before and after playing or working out.

Running

Tightness is the enemy here. You *gotta* stretch those legs out from heel to butt, front and back, preferably before and after.

Hamstring Stretch (page 34)
Downward Dog (page 35)
Standing Forward Bend (page 115)
Seated Forward Bend (page 117)

Biking

To compensate for the hunched-over position, it's important to stretch the muscles in the front of the chest and bend the lower spine in the opposite direction using:

Cat Stretch (page 19)
Triangle (page 90)
Cobra (page 12)
Bow (page 22)

Bow will also prevent tightness in the quads; for the hamstrings, see the prior running poses.

Tennis, Racquetball and Squash

Like golf, these are one-sided sports which can lead to muscular imbalances. Holding strength poses longer on the nondominant side and stretches longer on the strong side will help redress that. You also need full range of motion in your shoulder and elbow joints to prevent injury from the repetitive motion of the swing. That calls for:

Arms-Up Forward Bend (page 126)
Bow (page 22)

The legs take a pounding in the racket sports. To build strength and stability, try:

Warrior I, II and especially **III,** the **Airplane** variation (pages 49, 50, and 71).

Spinal twists enable and compensate for the corkscrew serving motion:

Kneeling Twist (page 25)
Seated Twist (page 24)

Swimming

The breathing exercises (pages 79–84) can really help you here. To stretch the upper back and maintain good range of motion in the shoulder and hip joints, practice:

Half Eagle (page 20)
Bow (page 22)
Triangle (page 90)
Pigeon (page 40)

To open up the whole front of your body and counteract swimming's forward- and downward-reaching motion, practice:

Wheel (page 57)

Basketball

Hoops means a lot of pounding on the hips and low back, due to all the jumping—or, really, the landings. So pay special attention to hip openers and hamstring stretchers.

Pigeon (page 40)
Downward Dog (page 35)
Hamstring Stretch (page 34)

Baseball and Softball

Hitting is all about hip turn, like the golf swing. That means:
Pigeon (page 40)
Warrior I (page 49)

Accelerating from home to first base (and hopefully, beyond) can wreak havoc on the hammies. Make sure to warm up overall first (**Sun Salutes**), then stretch 'em out with:

Downward Dog (page 35)
Standing Forward Bend (page 115)

Seated Forward Bend (page 117)

For full ROM in the throwing shoulder and limber back and arms:

Half Eagle (page 20)
Bow (page 22)
Cobra (page 12)
Arms-Up Forward Bend (page 126)

Hockey and Skating

All the poses that stretch the lower body will come into play here. More specifically, as with biking, you want to counter the forward-leaning posture with backbends and chest openers. This will not only help loosen the muscles but create the space you need to breathe properly and fully.

Cobra (page 12)
Bow (page 22)
Wheel (page 57)
Crescent Moon (page 37)

These sports also involve trunk rotation, so the twists are vital, as are the positions that stretch and strengthen the core—the muscles that support the trunk.

Kneeling Twist (page 25)
Seated Twist (page 24)
Triangle (page 90)

Skiing and Snowboarding

Positions that strengthen the legs, knee joints and lower back are key:

Warrior I, II, and III (pages 49, 50 and 71)
Triangle (page 90)

Seated Forward Bend (page 117)
Bridge (page 118)

Keep the legs flexible with:

Hamstring Stretch (page 34)
Downward Dog (page 35)

Balance poses are obviously great for the slopes:

Tree (page 65)
Eagle (page 68)
Warrior III (page 71)

Now that you understand and appreciate all the great physical benefits that come with regular posture and breath work, we're going to explore some exciting new yoga dimensions, ones that will take your performance to a whole new level. I'm talking about the mental and psychological edge that yoga gives any competitive athlete—and any competitive businessman. That is, the ability to focus, laserlike, on the task at hand and the power of deep relaxation, both of which allow you to tap your utmost potential and operate in The Zone.

Yoga Jocks

JOE INMAN

GOLFER, CHAMPIONS TOUR

Inman, 56, has won three tournaments on the Senior or Champions Tour and he's also a TV commentator. He took up yoga a couple of years back.

"Before I tried it I thought it was all those nuts from California who do yoga, people who want to be the Dalai Lama. But now I take classes about twice a week and I feel a difference in my body. It's wonderful. I wish to God I'd done this when I was 25. I'm sure I'm gonna do it for the rest of my life. Not just for golf, for life—I want to be the oldest living former Senior Tour player.

"Yoga's great for the mental game. My personality is too fast—my swing's too fast and my mind's too fast, too. When I'm doing TV, it's great, but on the course I'm constantly trying to slow down. In yoga you close your eyes and take deep breaths and consciously slow down, and I try to do that before a round, and even on the course—especially after two bogeys.

"When you're relaxed on the course, you still won't do everything right. But if you tense up, you have no chance. You just gotta hit it and let it go. Not everyone can do that. But the people who can't do that, you never heard of—they're not on the Tour."

The Real Man

MARTY STEIN

EXECUTIVE, TRADE ASSOCIATION, 53, ALEXANDRIA, VA

"In 1997, I was having some really nagging back problems. I was playing golf 3 to 4 times per week, and in order to play, I had to take 6 to 8 Advils—two before, two at the turn, two after—and I was wearing back braces for support.

"A masseuse convinced me to try yoga, and I went to around three classes per week and tried to do some every day and night at home. I immediately noticed a difference. I didn't put the brace on or take Advil, and at the end of the day I felt fine. And soon I could almost play every day if I wanted to.

"At the time, I was about a 10 to 12 handicap, and after I started practicing yoga, I got down to about a 7. Yoga allowed me to make a better turn. And having the strength in my legs and hams enabled me to have more stamina. When you come to the last few holes, if your legs get tired your swing gets lazy. Being stronger and more flexible helped me play more consistently.

"Before an important shot or during tournaments, walking from one ball to the next, I do deep breathing, a couple of good, deep yoga breaths. It has a calming effect. I also realized, that if I was in my car and got cut off, a couple of yoga breaths helped me from getting road rage and to just relax—it works in other aspects of my life, too."

CHAPTER 12
Staying Focused: Work Sharper, Play Better

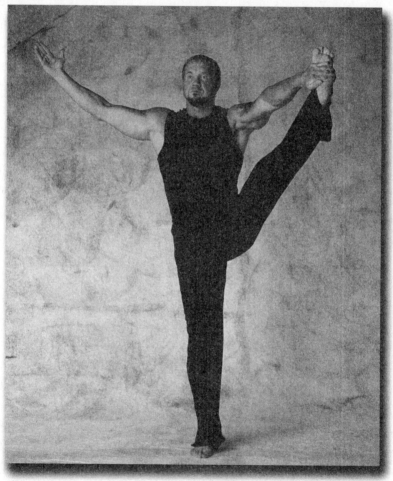

Balance poses and yoga in general trained wrestler Diamond Dallas Page to focus better. So much so that he overcame childhood learning disabilities and learned to read at a much higher level.

practice my breathing and focusing before every game," says **Kevin Garnett** of the Minnesota Timberwolves. "Yoga helps me calm down and helps me center my energy so I'm balanced instead of going out there and just spreading my energy all over the court. I'm zeroed in on the game and have my mind set on what I need to do."

If you follow sports at all, you know that this guy is an unbelievable basketball player, one of the top five in the NBA, which means in the world. Beyond his skills and talents, he also brings it every game, never taking a night off. That's consistent effort—and consistent focus. And he's been able to laser in like that ever since he came into the league straight outta *high school.*

Not coincidentally, that's when Garnett started practicing yoga. "I've been doing it since 1995. It's something I've liked ever since. It was difficult at times, but when you're young and you're spontaneous, you try all things. Fortunately I was able to carry it over to now." He explains that he does a full yoga workout in the off-season and during the grueling 82-game campaign, he just uses the breath work.

For Garnett and many other top athletes—see the sidebar on relief pitcher **Steve Reed** in this chapter—the breath is the vehicle that gets them mentally focused. First they block out everything but their respiration; then they transfer that complete attention to the task at hand. By making sure they are breathing fully and deeply, which we tend not to do in times of stress, they also ensure they're getting maximum oxygen intake, which helps them perform physically.

However, other yoga jocks say they're big believers in the yoga *poses* for honing their concentration. The attention and discipline the matwork requires trains them to bear down and be "in the moment" during games. **Kerry Kittles,** starting shooting guard for the New Jersey Nets, tried yoga before the 2001–2002 season when he was rehabbing from a knee operation. Along the way, Kerry noticed how yoga "helps your focus."

"Obviously playing professional sports is all about focus," he says. "And yoga's all about holding a pose and maintaining your focus on that, trying to get deeper and relaxing yourself at the same time. You do that for an hour-and-a-half session, three or four sessions a week, and you become better at keeping your mind on one thing and not letting your mind drift."

One area he specifically wanted to get better in was free throws. (He's a 78 percent career shooter at this writing, which is far from shabby. But not good enough for him.) "I have a tendency of not being focused while I'm at the line, so I try to think about the stuff that I did in yoga class to help me focus and relax when I am in a pose. It really helps you get where you want to be mentally," he says.

There's really no argument between these two groups of top performers; yoga breathing exercises and the positions *both* put you in a position to succeed—in sports and beyond.

For former WWE wrestler Diamond Dallas Page, focusing better via yoga has a whole different meaning, having nothing to do with body slams. When he was younger, Page had a lot of trouble with dyslexia and Attention Deficit Disorder. "I grew up not knowing how to read," he says. "You're talking about a guy who was 30 years old and reading at a third-grade level. Since I've gotten into yoga, the focus has really helped my reading big-time. I'm still not great, but I'm much better than I was."

To Page, being able to focus better ain't no game. And it's a serious business to David Cooke as well. An assistant district attorney in the Atlanta area, he prosecutes crimes against women and children: rapes, molestation, torture—the worst. Talk about pressure. "I'm in court almost every day fighting for justice," says Cooke, who's in his early 30s. "And if I lose, evil wins."

A 6'5" weight-lifter, boxer and kickboxer, Cooke started doing yoga in college. It helped him recover from knee surgery when traditional physical therapy wasn't working, and in the martial arts, he says, it gave him greater strength throughout his entire range of motion. But today he prizes yoga (breath work and poses) for the way it helps him stay focused during his criminal trials.

"The mental stress is very strong," he says, "but yoga helps me to be in the moment. When the judge is chewing my ass out and the defense attorney is cheating, I need to address what's happening *now;* not the last battle I already lost or the next battle, either."

During a recent trial, Cooke noticed that "I was doing yoga breathing, deep breathing in and out, through the nose. And it helped me to remain calm. Like when you're in Downward Dog, you're not thinking about Warrior, just in breath, out breath, your hamstrings . . . You're completely in that moment."

As you've just heard, the body and breath work we're already doing will greatly improve your ability to focus, on and off the playing field. Here's a new, additional exercise that will specifically train your concentration even more. It's a balance pose, probably the best kind for developing focus, and this one requires you to balance on the smallest body part yet: your toes. (You'll feel right away that this move has a pretty intense strength component, too, working the front of your shins as well as stretching the muscles in your feet, ankles and thighs.)

TOE BALANCE

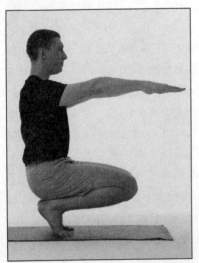

◆ Hunker down on the mat with your hands on the floor in front of you. Raise yourself up on the balls of your feet, then:

◆ Inhale and bring your torso erect, lifting your hands off the floor. Now you are balancing only on the toes, thighs roughly parallel with the floor. Find your balance with your hands resting on the tops of your knees and then extend your arms straight out. Breathe.

◆ After 5 full breaths, try to move your knees, which should be close together, down even closer to the floor. This will rock your torso back a little and push you up even farther up on your toes, requiring another balance adjustment.

◆ When you're stable again, you can raise your arms up to the prayer position in the front of your chest (optional).

◆ Break the pose by rocking back on your heels.

Working this narrow edge is kinda tricky, no? It requires full concentration, and that's the point. After you've done this 2 or 3 times to get the hang of the form, try these variations, both of which also require intense focus, but in slightly different ways:

◆ Repeat, but this time, try to keep your attention on your breath, not your body, its movements, or the balance challenge you're engaged in. Focus on making each inhale and exhale full and deliberate. Do for 10 full breaths, then come down.

Notice any difference in how you feel, or how well you were able to do the exercise? Were you able to focus on your breath throughout, or did you jump back and forth between that and making sure you stayed on your toes?

In this last variation, we'll ratchet up the degree of difficulty and turn the focus inward at the same time. How? Simply:

◆ Repeat the **Toe Balance**, with eyes closed. Or try to anyway—this is a toughie.

I recommend using this eyes-closed focus exercise as an extra, occasional supplement to your regular balance work. When you want to emphasize focus a little more—or change things up for variety's sake—sub this in for one of the other balance poses in our rookies and veterans workouts, and try it all three ways. Or, if you really like this one, go ahead and add it in permanently.

Yoga Jocks

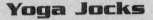

STEVE REED

RELIEF PITCHER, COLORADO ROCKIES

Reed is one of baseball's top "set-up" men, the one-inning specialists who enter the game when the opposing team is rallying—his whole job is dealing with high-pressure situations. To help him concentrate and come through in the clutch, he turns to yogic breathing techniques.

"When I first approach the mound, I just try to take one exaggerated breath and blow it out. Just try and slow my breathing down. The tendency is to want to speed things up, to get the ball back faster, to throw the next pitch faster and thinking, 'Let's get out of this,' instead of slowing down and having command over the things I can control, and that's making the next pitch. When I go out there and I take my last deep breath, it kind of locks me in.

"I block out all the things that are going through my mind: There are runners on second and third, it's a one-run game, I haven't been pitching good, I got in an argument with my wife. That's what the breathing does; it keeps me in the moment, with *this pitch.* Then, when I get the ball back, I try to control the next pitch.

"It works for me; in pressure situations I've been able to perform better because of these techniques. A lot of guys have the playing ability, but not the mental side. I feel this gives me a little bit of an advantage. And it's been a calming influence, not just in baseball, but also in my personal life."

CHAPTER 13

Deep Relaxation: Stress Busting & the Best Sleep of Your Life

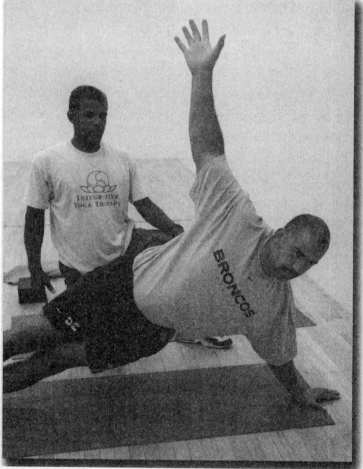

Hal Stoelzle/*Rocky Mountain News*, 2000

Yoga trainer Danny Poole, rear, reminds NFL lineman Lester Archambeau to keep his facial muscles relaxed. "Don't geek up. Soften the face and breathe. . . . " We'll use a similar de-stressing technique at the end of this chapter.

From the minute you begin your first real yoga workout, you will start relaxing your body and mind. The stretching releases built-up muscle and body tension, alignment improves and blood flow increases, oxygenating and restoring your whole system. This is why you hear so many guys marvel at how great they felt after their *very first* yoga session, before they even knew what they were doing!

That yoga glow—the "just feels great" effect I alluded to at the very beginning of the book—is a gift that keeps on giving. Guys like it so much, they get hooked; you often hear them say, "It's like I'm addicted to yoga; my body wants to feel that good again."

Bob Eriksen, 52, is a real estate developer and construction guy out in California. He took up yoga in 2002; his doctor "prescribed" it for him when he was recovering from the last of three knee surgeries. He's such a convert that he goes to 4 to 5 morning classes a week. "You get a glow from it from the A.M. all the way to the evening," he says. "I feel like I have better circulation, like my body's waking up. . . . You feel normal, right, the way you should."

The happy yoga addicts will tell you that the relaxation they feel is both physical and mental. The two are really inseparable, anyway, maybe even identical. When your body feels good, you feel good. When you feel good mentally, your body will almost always go along for the ride. And studies bear out that yoga works to de-stress you from both ends at once.

In a Japanese study published in 2000, seven yoga instructors were monitored during exercise. Two important stress-related changes were observed. One, alpha waves—the kind of brain activity seen during sleep and deep relaxation—increased. Two, serum cortisol—a steroid hormone produced in times of stress—decreased. Another recent study done in India shows that both body and mind are relieved. In it, 20 patients with mild to moderate hypertension, aged 35 to 55, did yoga one hour a day for three months. The results included decreased blood pressure as well as lowered cholesterol and triglycerides. And on the psychological front, the subjects reported "overall improvement in subjective well-being and quality of life."

The yogic focus on deeper, regular breathing is definitely a factor in reducing tension as well. (What do people say you should do when you're having a freak-out moment? Take a deep breath, right?) Another theory that has both yoga folks and Western medical people behind it has to do with the sympathetic and parasympathetic nervous systems.

These are two complementary parts of your autonomic nervous system. The sympathetic system gets excited, revving the body up to confront danger or outside stresses by raising your heart rate and releasing energy and adrenaline, among other things—the classic fight-or-flight response. The parasympathetic basically does the opposite, sending its own neurotransmitters to slow your heart rate, etc., calming you down. This network is also thought to promote healing, sleep and digestion, plus help maintain a healthy reproductive system.

The sympathetic system's impulses seem to originate in the thoracic and lumbar areas of the spine; the para's originate in the brain stem and/or the sacral spine. (Eastern medicine's explanation for soothing feelings emanating from that spot is that there's a major chakra or energy center there.)

The stress hormones secreted by the sympathetic system have long-term corrosive or degenerative effects. (Being angry all the time doesn't just *feel* bad—it *is* bad for you.) As the study I cited showed, yoga dampens down that response. Even better news: Yoga seems to turn on the parasympathetic system, calming and relaxing the body. John Douillard, author of *Mind, Body and Sport,* thinks it has to do with nose-breathing rather than mouth-breathing. Others cite the activation of the diaphragm in deep yogic breathing, and still others point to the deep stretching as the trigger mechanism for the feel-good system.

Whatever the exact mechanism, it works. This helps explain why guys who've been doing yoga for a while often find that they are calmer and happier. Not just not just on the mat or right after a yoga workout, but in their entire lives. Take Bob Hagg, the fire captain we heard from before who said that yoga helped prevent injuries to his men. In addition, he says, yoga has taken some of the stress out of their high-pressure, dangerous occupation. "I sleep better," he notes. "We all sleep better. And I know my stress level was reduced. In the stressful situations, it's your attitude that's different. Little things that bother other people don't bother us. Physically, mentally . . . we've been doing it for so long now that it's just routine to us, but other people see it in us and remark on it."

As much as NHLer **Sean Burke** appreciates what yoga's done for him as a hockey player, he's also amazed at what it's done for him off the ice. "The first year and a half after I started yoga, I just felt good all the time," he says. "I could definitely notice the difference. I still feel pretty good now, but I probably noticed it more before. Maybe it's changed me to the point where this is how I'm *supposed* to be. My demeanor is so much better. I don't get angry. It takes a lot to piss me off now, and I couldn't say that about myself in the past."

De-stressing with yoga doesn't stop when your waking hours end. Another great relaxation benefit that yoga guys swear by is:

GETTING THE BEST SLEEP OF YOUR LIFE

Bob Eriksen, our Mr. Feelgood from above, says that since he's been doing yoga: "I sleep sounder, but actually get up earlier. I just need 6 to 7 hours a night because my body is performing optimally, so smoothly, and I'm getting so much energy from the yoga. Before I used to try to get 8 to 10 hours, but now I can't sleep that much; I'm up and ready to go."

Of course, you don't want to get too calm, and lose your competitive edge. The last thing you want is to get so mellow that you become passive, happily snoozing through life while other guys are eating your lunch. Not to worry. Being calm under pressure is a big part of getting and staying focused. That combo allows you to function better, to achieve your goals easier—even if your goal is to go out and kick some butt!

When Peter Scirios, a 47-year-old architect in San Luis Obispo, California, was playing semi-pro rugby, yoga helped with all the bruises and injuries. But it certainly didn't interfere with his ability to compete—in fact, it enhanced it with a cold-blooded clarity of mind. "I was able to deal with pre-game adrenaline rushes and all the anxiousness," he says. "The breathing allowed me to handle that better. Instead of an aggressive freak-out, you can go out there with what I would call an aggressive calmness."

Right now we can begin to consciously cultivate our defenses against stress and continue to practice our concentration in the same simple exercise. Try this right after you finish your next workout—yoga or whatever. (Make sure the surroundings are quiet and conducive to relaxing.) This might sound contradictory, but we're going to very purposefully and intentionally chill out. And the de-stressing, after only 5 minutes, can be very, very powerful.

5-MINUTE RELAXATION

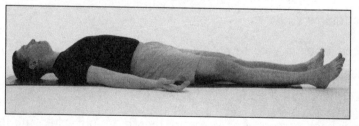

◆ Lie back on the floor or mat and stretch out. Let the arms and hands fall naturally to the sides and arrange your legs however they're comfortable. In Yoga-ese, this is known as *Shavasana,* or Corpse Pose, if that helps you get the picture. Without getting too morbid about it, you just want to lie there motionless.

◆ Close your eyes and keep them closed throughout. Take 5 long, slow breaths, trying to fully fill and empty your lungs (without forcing or overdoing it). If your breath is still speeded up from working out, take as many slow breaths as you need to get back to deliberate breathing.

◆ Now we're going to consciously relax every part of your body, starting with your left foot. Put your attention on it and, without moving the foot or changing your breathing (or opening your eyes), just think about your left foot becoming completely relaxed. You might say silently to yourself: "Left foot relaxed . . ."

◆ Move your attention up a little to the left ankle and think of that joint entering its most relaxed state possible. "Left ankle relaxed." Pause briefly to let your message to the body sink in. Throughout you can also, if you like, imagine on your inhales that you are actually sending oxygen to the area you intend to relax.

◆ Continue through the left calf, left knee, left thigh and left hip.

◆ Start over with the right foot and move up through the hip.

◆ Relax the arms, starting with the left fingers, hand, then left forearm, left upper arm and shoulder. Repeat on the right. Keep the breath slow and even.

◆ Concentrate on your lower back, sending it the signal to relax fully. Since this is such a trouble area for many guys, you might want to linger here a little longer and repeat the message.

◆ Upper back relaxed. Let the entire length of your back sink into the floor; you want to lie completely flat.

◆ Now relax the belly, observing it gently rise and fall with your breath. Relax the chest.

◆ Relax the throat and neck, front and back, focusing in your mind's eye on those areas and visualizing them letting go of whatever tension might be held there.

◆ Relax the face muscles. It helps to first make an exaggerated grimace, scrunching your facial muscles, making lines in the forehead and tightening the throat cords—then releasing it all at once and letting your face lie quiet. Imagine your eyes sinking deeper into their sockets, completely loose and at rest.

◆ Finally, imagine any tension that still remains in your body escaping through the very top of your head. Try doing this on an exhale, so you are expelling a breath and the lingering stress at the same time.

◆ Return your attention to your breath (it may well be slower by now). Follow it for 5 complete breaths, then when you are ready, open your eyes.

You might be amazed at what just 5 minutes of "doing nothing" can do. If you doubt that just thinking or visualizing can really effect physiological changes in your body, I have two words for you:

"Sexual fantasies."

See what I mean? Just thinking certain thoughts—you know which ones I'm talking about—can cause a whole set of demonstrable effects in the male body, changing respiration, temperature and making a truly remarkable difference in blood flow. That's the power of visualization and concentration.

Now we're going to learn how to take the focus and relaxation we've studied in the last two chapters up to even higher, rarer levels. To get there, we're going to try a little meditation. Like everything in this book, it's strictly optional; if you're not comfortable with this idea right now, walk away. Maybe you'll come back to it later.

But let me just say that meditation is simple, easy and it's been scientifically proven to yield tremendous benefits, beyond those you can get from yoga alone. So what have you got to lose? Well, I'll tell you what's at stake, what you're risking here: 15 minutes.

I think that's a risk you can afford to take. Believe me, the payoff is worth it. To give you an idea, the first guy we're going to hear from in the next section is Oakland A's pitcher **Barry Zito,** one of the best pitchers in baseball. And he meditates before every game.

The Real Man
TED ROMAN

BUILDING CONTRACTOR, 53, ROYAL OAK, MICHIGAN

"Two years ago my doctor told me I had prostate cancer and needed radiation. I started doing some reading and I didn't like the odds and side effects of what he wanted to do. I started changing my eating habits and I tried yoga. I lost a lot of weight and haven't felt this good in my life.

"I'm still working; I'm in the sheet metal business. Guys I work with go: 'Yeah, right, you're in there chanting.' They don't know that it's a real workout.

"I go six days a week and it gets me through having cancer. The only time I don't think about it is when I'm there. It's important to relieve stress, and the practice carries me during the day. If you find you're not thinking about the right things, you can do some breathing and relax.

"It makes me calmer. And I actually sleep more. I slept four hours per night and now I sleep more and feel better. A lot of my new outlook is from yoga. The rat race isn't as important as taking care of yourself. I even get along better with my ex-wife because I don't have all that hostility and it helped me let all that stuff go."

CHAPTER 14
Meditation: Going Deeper Within

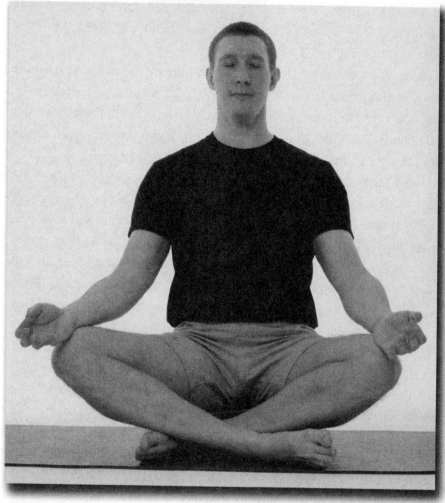

©Erica Berger, 2003

Breath awareness meditation sounds simple enough to do: "Don't move and don't think." You'll find, though, that it's a challenging task, one that brings profound and positive results.

Before a recent game against the Devil Rays in St. Petersburg, Florida, most of the Oakland A's were talking, listening to music, playing cards or working on crossword puzzles in the visitors' locker room. Pitcher **Barry Zito** sat on a stool in front of his locker, then casually extended his right leg skyward to his right hand, looking like a NFL punter. "A move like this would have been impossible for me before yoga," he said. "Flexibility-wise, I was struggling. My hammies were tight, my groin was tight. My hips have really benefited."

Zito, 25, was among the first athletes to hook up with Los Angeles conditioning guru Alan Jaeger, in 1998. The results have been nothing short of phenomenal. In 2002, just his third year in the majors, the left-hander won the American League Cy Young award, given to the best pitcher of that season, after compiling a 23–5 record.

Obviously there's more to his success than yoga, but Zito gives his mat work major credit—no matter what some of his lunkhead peers might think. "Some guys might think of it as feminine and give you grief about it," he says. "But any athlete who laughs at yoga is essentially mocking the fact that the body needs to be loose and physically strong—and strong in certain positions, which is what yoga is. Plus, if your body is stretched out, loose, strong and flexible and you keep yourself hydrated, the chance of injury decreases greatly."

Yoga's also a big part of Zito's mental game—and his competitive edge. He's made meditation an integral part of his pre-game ritual. By the time the 6'4", 215-pound hurler heads to the mound, he appears to be almost in a trance. "We athletes need to be in touch with ourselves mentally to do the crazy stuff we do out there," he says. "Knowing relaxation techniques helps calm you down, which is very important on the mound. It's definitely a mental cleanser. Yoga brings the physical, mental and spiritual together, and not a lot of other exercise methods do that."

He's hooked, but you may still have questions about meditation. Like: *Is meditation yoga?*

Absolutely. In fact, some yoga experts say that the original purpose of all the *asanas* (poses) and *pranayama* (breath work) was to get the body loose enough and the mind calm enough to sit still in meditation.

That being said, you can certainly practice yoga without meditating. And that's certainly an option in the way you use this book. My view, though, is that you'd be missing out. Meditating is a distilled form of yoga's focus and relaxation work—and the results can be even more powerful. It has a profoundly positive and relaxing effect, a great counter to daily life anxiety. But as we've also heard from Mr. Zito, this intense, purposeful form of deep relaxation energizes you, too, and prepares you to go out and function at your best. Look at it this way: Just like some of the variations on poses we've been learning, meditation Super-Charges yoga.

Sounds good, but I still don't see: What is it?

Meditation is essentially a period of concentrated relaxation, a turning of your focus inward that later helps you deal with the world outside. The goal is to become as completely aware of where you are and what you are doing as possible, including the state of your body and the functioning of your breath. To accomplish this, you basically concentrate on your breath, an object or a word, called a mantra—a neutral subject that you focus on intently, to the exclusion of everything else.

Is meditation a religious thing?

Not the way we're going to do it. Like the way we're approaching yoga overall in this book, our take on meditation is basically utilitarian; it's just a tool to be used. Lots of guys we respect say it benefits them. There's science that says it's beneficial, too. So let's just see if it works for you.

Meditation is indeed very personal and private (though you can do it in a group). Is it spiritual, as Zito describes it? Well, I would say that it honors and nurtures your spirit, and if you believe that you are a part of anything bigger and more cosmic than your carpool in this life, then it honors that, and maybe even gets you in closer contact with it.

Okay, how do I do it?

The most bare-bones definition or instruction I can think of is this: Don't move and don't think. Still tough to picture, right? So why don't we just try it right now, and afterward, we'll explore more how it benefits you and the ways science says meditation achieves all that it does.

BREATH-AWARENESS MEDITATION

This method reinforces yoga's focus on the breath, and I find it easier than some other techniques. For example, when I've tried concentrating on a word or mantra, repeating it silently to myself over and over while meditating, I find I inevitably begin to dwell on the meaning of that word, and as you'll see, we don't want to dwell.

◆ Find a quiet place and turn down the lights. Pitch-dark can be too conducive to sleep, so I'd keep some soft light on. Turn off the phone, make sure you won't be disturbed.

◆ You can meditate in any position really, but lying down is a sure ticket to snooze-land. So I recommend sitting down, either cross-legged on the floor, as you've traditionally seen it, or sitting in a chair that keeps your back straight (that facilitates the flow of air). Chair or not, don't slouch. Your entire body should be relaxed; get yourself comfortable, then try not to move any more. You may find it helpful to do the **5-Minute Relaxation** we just learned.

◆ Rest your hands lightly on your thighs or knees. Traditionally you're taught to touch your thumbs to your forefingers, closing an energy circuit. So try that or not; just don't clench your fists.

◆ Close your eyes part way or all the way. If you leave them half-open, look out at the ground a little ways in front of you and keep a very soft focus on that area. But don't stare at it or scrutinize it.

◆ Turn your attention to your breath. Two ways to follow it are a) focus on the sensations of air coming into and leaving your nostrils or b) follow the in-and-out movement of your belly as you exhale and inhale. (I'm a nose man myself.)

◆ Now follow the breath in and out, putting all your conscious attention on its ebb and flow without altering it. Just monitor it, note it. As you get deeper into the meditation, you will probably find that your breathing pattern is slowing down. That's fine, just notice it. But don't try to consciously slow down, let it happen (if it does). Continue to follow the breath.

◆ Resist the temptation to move. Even if you get an itch, see if you can wait it out instead of yielding to it and scratching. Just let your attention go to the itchy place, note to yourself that it itches, then return your attention to your breath. It's surprising how often the itch will give up and go away once you decide you're not playing its game. Same for mild aches and pains. Obviously if you start to have severe pain somewhere, give yourself a break. No bed-of-nails martyrdom here, please.

◆ Do this for 5 minutes the first time out. Then simply open your eyes all the way. Now try to remember what it was like to be really still. That will help you return to that state. Purposely take control of your breath now, and breathe really deeply. Moving slowly at first, stretch out, shake out your limbs—and scratch anywhere you want. You may feel like you're awakening from a deep sleep; in fact, meditation has been shown to confer all the benefits of sleep in a much shorter time. Just a few minutes can refresh you like an hour's nap.

I know, I know: You kept having thoughts, you couldn't stay focused on your breath. Don't worry; meditation only seems simple. Doing it is incredibly complicated. Many people find it easier to stay focused if they count their breaths as they happen. To do this, on the first exhale, say "One" to yourself, then do the same for breaths (exhales) "Two," "Three" and "Four." Then start over. When you lose count, as you inevitably will, just start over at one. This seems to give your mind—frantic to be doing something, race around and think about a hundred things at once—enough to do so that it will calm down, but is not so distracting that it disrupts your concentration.

That's the tricky part. While you may be able to sit still, your mind doesn't want to. Or at least it's been habituated to go a million miles a minute and keep churning out thoughts like widgets on an assembly line. That frantic stream-of-consciousness or interior monologue is what we are trying to interrupt and counteract by meditating. This is the "Don't Think" part of the "Don't Move, Don't Think" instruction I gave you earlier. And it's harder than you might . . . think.

In fact, you may never succeed. That's right, you may never be able to banish thoughts completely; even the most experienced meditators can only do that for short periods of time. The goal, then, is to let go of thinking as much as you can, and by really seeing how much your mind is occupied by these thoughts, noting them as they come up, it gives you distance from them.

You come to understand—and this is key—that you are not your thoughts. You have them; *don't let them have you.* In the long run, this will diminish the power of your thoughts—especially negative thoughts—to change your mood. Being able to recognize when you are having negative thoughts that, "These thoughts are not me. They are just some thoughts I'm having" is an incredibly liberating thing.

So when you catch yourself thinking during meditation, just note it silently to yourself. You could say simply "I'm thinking" or "I'm thinking about tonight's dinner," or whatever it might be. Just note that you're thinking, then return to following the breath. Don't try to suppress the thoughts or deny they are happening. That won't work; since they *are* happening, you'll just be in denial and you'll lose the intimate connection with what's going on with yourself right then. And that defeats the whole purpose of "being in the moment." But you also don't have to get caught up in your thoughts.

You might want to try this technique that Danny Poole teaches the University of Colorado football team for dealing with thoughts that come up. "Some people say, 'Let it go,'" he says. "But how the hell do you do that? And you're gonna think. So I don't tell 'em 'Don't think.'" Instead, he says, "Acknowledge what comes up, thank it for coming up, and tell it you'll take care of it later." Then, Poole says, you dismiss that thought "with a firm but gentle 'Bye.'"

"We all have concerns, that's natural," he elaborates. "So just say, 'Hey, thanks for coming up, my concern. I look forward to dealing with that, but right now I'm focusing or I'm resting. So, Bye.'"

This also comes in handy when you are having a tough time getting to sleep. Poole's seen with his athletes that the night before games can be particularly tough. "You can toss and turn, thinking about the fact that the game's on ESPN, your parents are coming and you're hoping their tickets will be ready for them. Then you're going over your game assignments in your mind. Just accept they came up and tell 'em bye."

For most readers, the pre-game anxiety might come the night before a big business meeting. "I work with an attorney who's using this," says Poole. "When he's thinking about trials in bed at night, he does the same thing." Having tried this, I think it's very effective during meditation, too. See if it works for you.

The point is: Get away from your thoughts and back to the breath. It might also help when detaching from a thought to say this silently to yourself: "Back to the breath." Don't get mad at yourself for being a thought machine. We all are. Besides, getting mad doesn't do any good. Some Eastern philosophers refer to this all-too-human tendency as "puppy mind." Our minds run here and there and side to side, sniffing everything, easily distracted. So you give your mind a gentle tug on the leash and tell it to get back on the sidewalk and move forward. When dealing with minds as with puppies, positive reinforcement gets you a lot further than negative.

Now that we know how it's done, lets get back to answering some other questions about meditating. Like:

How does this help me?

It's only logical that practicing being "present" or "in the moment" like this can help you in sports or high-pressure job situations where a moment—a split second—is all you have to react properly. Los Angeles Lakers coach **Phil Jackson** has famously used meditation to win nine NBA championships.

Less obvious, however, is just how meditation relieves anxiety and stress and delivers a profound sense of well-being to those who practice consistently. Yet a long tradition, a world of anecdotal evidence and some fascinating research tell us that it's so.

One component that makes a lot of sense to me—and that feels right, given my meditation experience—has to do with the nature of anxiety. So much of the stress and worry that we carry with us has to do with a) things that happened in the past that we didn't like and b) the fear that past badness (or some fresh disaster, embarrassment or pain) might happen in the future. We carry these twin preoccupations around—and what happens to the present? It disappears, in effect, because we are mentally living in the future or the past.

When you are consciously in the moment—a time when, odds are, nothing that bad is happening—it helps you break those negative thought patterns and provides a huge amount of stress relief. If you want to work on this, you try this out: As you settle in to meditate (or, really, anytime you want to emphasize the positive) say to yourself, "There is absolutely nothing wrong with this moment." It makes you realize that you are having some "quality time," so to speak, you've found a quiet relaxing time in your life to meditate or enjoy. More than that, though, it makes you realize just how *many* moments there are in every day that are really pretty excellent—if you're living them and not stuck in the past or sweating the future. When bad moments occur, and they will, this perspective will also help you deal more effectively with problems and move on, making it less likely they will keep returning to haunt you mentally.

Here's a personal tip that might help reinforce being present for you: Sometimes when I sit down to meditate, for the first few breaths I'll say to myself, "Right here . . . right now." The first part goes with the inhale, the second on the exhale. It's just a reminder of where I am and that this particular slice of time counts. In fact, I sometimes use this when I'm not meditating. For instance, I've been walking on the beach on Long Island with my wife on a beautiful day and found myself dwelling on all kinds of unrelated things. When I catch myself, I'll say "Right here, right now" to remind myself to be in the moment—and enjoy it for all it's worth.

On a physiological level, we're just beginning to understand how meditation does what it does. One way is by making changes in the brain. In January of 2003, the *Wall Street Journal*—no hippy-dippy New Age publication—reported that Professor Richard Davidson of the University of Wisconsin gave 23 subjects meditation training once a week for eight weeks. Another 16 subjects, a control group, got no training. After the eight weeks the researchers saw that brain activity had shifted in the meditators so there were more neurons firing in the left side of the frontal cortex than in the right. "That pattern is associated with positive feelings such as joy, happiness and low levels of anxiety," explained reporter Sharon Begley. The nonmeditating group showed no such shift, and the positive results of the meditating group were confirmed again 16 weeks later.

Another feel-good explanation comes from a Danish study that showed that the release of dopamine—the neurotransmitter involved in the brain's regulation of emotional responses and pleasure—increased up to 65 percent during meditation.

There's also some evidence that the deep breathing in meditation is a benefactor when it comes to mood-improvement. Research done in Italy recently looked at two groups of people: one reciting Ave Marias (this was Italy, after all); the other meditating and reciting a mantra. The summary of findings noted that for both groups, "rhythm formulas that involve breathing at six breaths a minute induce favorable psychological and possibly physiological effects."

Meditators often say they sleep better, and there's scientific backup for that, too. An Australian study published in *Biological Psychology* in 2000 showed significantly higher levels of melatonin on nights after subjects meditated versus nights without meditating. Melatonin is the naturally occurring hormone that some people take in an over-the-counter supplement as a sleeping aid, especially to fight jet lag.

The science is completely credible, but guys who meditate don't need studies to believe. They're sure. Let's check back in with David Cooke, the assistant district attorney in Atlanta we heard from earlier. He swears that yogic meditation has really had a profound and positive impact on his life.

Talk about stress. Remember, he prosecutes horrible crimes against women and children. "It really gets to us," he says. "I'm very conscious of how my job affects my blood pressure and my health. I have to undo what I'm doing to myself every day. Plus I've got two kids in diapers at home right now, so it's a lot to deal with."

That's why, Cooke says, "I've recently returned more to yoga, even if I can only do 10 minutes a night. And when I can, I do 30 to 60 minutes; that's gravy." After the poses, Cooke does some meditation, which he combines with Christian prayer. "What I do is based in the breath," he says, "the inhale and exhale, the breath of life. It creates a restful time, when I say, 'Thank you Lord for your help.'

"I gotta tell you, it's so beneficial. By the time you're done, basically your problems look a lot smaller. I'm able to deal with the child stuff at work better. And taking this time is a cue for me to de-stress, I associate it in my head with calming down. It means it's time to stop worrying and go to bed."

Cooke doesn't see any contradiction between his religious beliefs and his yoga practice. In fact, they reinforce each other. "I'm a Baptist, not a Hindu," he says. "But to me, if something's good it's a gift from God. I don't care what religion it's related to."

Remember when I said early on that the guys you think do yoga aren't really the guys who do yoga? David Cooke is living proof. "I grew up in the South, in the sticks—I'm the last guy you can be prejudiced against." (I think he's saying he's a redneck.) "If I can get into yoga," he says, "anyone can. Look—if you can take aspirin, take vitamins, why can't you do this other thing that's available that's so fantastic for your mental and physical health? It's so far beyond going to some gym; this is the best exercise for total health. Maybe some guys are afraid they're gonna get a red dot on their head or something. . . . For the life of me, I can't figure out why more people don't do yoga."

DEVELOPING YOUR OWN MEDITATION PRACTICE

Try sitting for 5 minutes at first, then work up to 10, then 15 as you feel ready. Eventually go for 20. Thirty rocks, but 20 seems to be long enough for the benefits of meditation to kick in, without it becoming a marathon test of your will and patience. You want to keep doing this, so don't make it too hard at first.

You can keep time by setting an alarm, using an egg timer, or just opening your eyes when you think the right time has elapsed. Or you could ask your wife to come and knock when the time is up. I suggest a timer of some kind, though, so you don't keep interrupting yourself and sneaking peeks at the clock.

People who do this every day really swear by that routine; some even do it once in the A.M. and once in the evening. For me, it's tough to find that kind of time—or maybe it's hard for me to maintain that kind of discipline. Either way, I shoot for 3 times a week, on the days that I don't do yoga (I count that as a mini-meditation). You'll work out your own best routine if you decide to keep meditating at all. But I urge you to give it a good shot.

CHAPTER 15
The Payoff:
Peak Performance
in The Zone

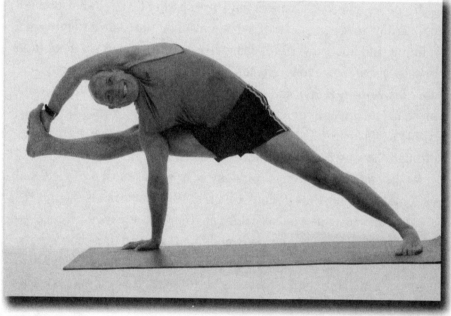

As Michael Lechonczak demonstrates here, yoga doesn't just expand your capabilities; it also prepares you to perform in a deeply focused state of flow. Not just in yoga, but in any sport you play.

At this point, you've seen it all. One by one, we've worked our way through all the physical and mental benefits yoga delivers. Call 'em the Big Six: Flexibility, Strength, Balance, Breathing, Focus and Relaxation. We've seen how yoga prevents injuries and how specific poses work best for certain sports. And we've begun to study how meditation can raise those last two benefits to even higher levels, paying dividends in all areas of your life.

If you've hung with me this far, I'm guessing that you may already be starting to get a sense of what's available to you through yoga training, and how powerful it can really be. That makes it a good time to talk about how your greater awareness and increased physical abilities work *together* and build on each other. Again, I don't want to sound too whole-grainy, but it's *synergistic*. Or as Michael L. would say, it's an "upward spiral," positive things that get even better through the way they build on each other.

At the end of that positive spiral is one of yoga's most profound, and in some ways most mysterious benefits. What happens is that all the abilities and insights you've gained in your private yoga practice go with you as you move your body and mind outward to perform in the public world. They're still there, sitting in you like an inexhaustible bank account. But you no longer need to focus your conscious attention on them to draw on them. You just know with an absolute certainty that your body's skills and your mind's judgment can prevail no matter what the demands. So all you have to do is focus on the current task, be it a golf swing, returning a blazing tennis serve, making a catch and throwing home in baseball, or finishing a road race.

When you can act and react like that—unconsciously, intuitively, in the flow—you're in The Zone, the land of peak performance. You've probably experienced this at some point, and you've heard athletes talk about playing in this ideal state. What you may not have realized is: Yoga gets you there.

Here's how it works:

While you were putting your body into all these new positions, you had to concentrate, to be very conscious of exactly what all your body parts were doing at each given moment. And, if your experience was like mine when I started yoga, you were surprised and gratified to see all the different ways you could move, twist, stretch, fold and bend. Plus, through these new challenges, I realized just how strong I really am. Yoga was also the first time that I ever really thought about—and understood—how I breathe in different situations. All of these things give you greater body awareness.

This awareness deepens as time goes on; the more you explore, the more you learn. **Eddie George** has been doing yoga for five-plus years now, which probably makes him the dean of Yoga Jocks. "After five years," he says, "you really get to know your body, know your weaknesses and strengths, how strong you are, how lazy you are. . . . You learn what you need to do to relax and breathe, and you find out how far you can push yourself. I got into yoga for flexibility, but after a while I realized that it's really about coming to yourself and finding out about yourself."

It only makes sense—when you study something as closely as you scrutinize your body in yoga, over time, you see things that you wouldn't otherwise notice. "You get more intimate with your body, real intimate," says Alan Jaeger, the West Coast baseball yoga guru. "A guy just stretching out his hamstring may or may not be paying attention or learning anything about his body. But when you spend 2 hours a day, 4 to 7 days a week, doing yoga like we do in our camp, you're really getting to know your body well and how it works.

"Think about it like this: If you hang out with a girl for a week, you might get to know her some, but if you hang out with her for a year, every day, you will get to know her on a completely different level."

Hey, wait a minute. We guys spend a lot of time and energy avoiding intimacy, and here I am promoting it. All this "getting in touch with" stuff sounds like a Sensitive Guy routine, doesn't it? And I promised you that this yoga book wouldn't be like that.

Not to worry. Body awareness just means getting in touch with yourself, your own male body, and finding out how capable you really are—by yourself and for your own benefit. We're cool with that, right? Right.

Once you have improved body awareness, you then develop greater body control. Nick Cardillicchio, the New York photographer who took up yoga after September 11, says: "Now I can engage and feel every muscle in my body, from my biceps to my quads. I can even isolate and flex the left side of my left foot."

The goal, of course, is not just to be able to twitch a few toes at will but to use this new body control, putting it to work helping you accomplish your tasks and goals. For Cardillicchio, that happens on photo shoots. "I really use my body in my work," he says. "Often I'll find myself hanging halfway upside down from a catwalk or standing with one foot on a ladder to get a certain shot. And it used to be difficult or leave me in pain." Now, Nick says, he understands better how he can position his body to get the shot without putting himself at risk. And thanks to the flexibility, strength and balance work he's put in, he's *able* to position himself in optimal ways.

Greater body control will clearly enhance performance in any sport. Think about the ultra-thin line in golf, the tiny differences in motion that make the difference between hitting it right and hitting it wrong. And then trying to hit it right the same way, time after time. That's body control. Eddie George's task is rougher but really no less complex: running the football and avoiding tackles. "Because I know my body better and what it can do," he says, "I'm more elusive now."

Knowledge is power. In this context, that means that greater understanding of your body through yoga gives you better control over it, and that in turn expands your body's capabilities. Don't forget, though, that power is power, too. With yoga you're not just more aware of your body and its abilities, you're also *improving* them, extending your physical limits through the work that you do in the poses. And as your capabilities grow, your awareness grows right along with it. Now you'll be able to recognize (or invent) more and different ways to exploit your newly expanded skills, which will in turn expand them even further, and so on. Like I said, the resulting whole is greater than the sum of its parts.

Gaining this new power is a great feeling, and you don't have to practice yoga very long to get it. Right from the start, I bet you'll discover abilities that you never knew you had, and that's a really pleasing surprise. Then you'll start to see improvement, and it's very gratifying to get better at something as demanding and complex as yoga.

However, there's another step in this evolution, the ultimate stage of yoga synergy. Not everyone gets there; this level requires greater abilities and a greater commitment to yoga. Beyond this synergy of body awareness and body control there's body mastery, or as sports scientists call it, proprioception.

BODY MASTERY AND WHAT THE HECK IS PROPRIOCEPTION?

As your intimacy—whoops, I mean your familiarity—with your body expands, and you see your capabilities improve. Says Alan Jaeger, "You are making a very powerful connection." Through it you are able to build what he calls "deep trust." It's complete confidence in your body; from all you've done to prepare it with yoga and other forms of training, you just *know* that it will respond well to any challenge. "It can scare men sometimes to say, 'I'm in touch with my body,'" says Eric Paskel of Sanga Yoga. "But it's really about learning how to honor yourself and have faith in your system to perform for you."

Having that faith frees you, the athlete, from having to think about what your body is doing or consciously trying to make it respond—it just does it by itself. This body mastery, the ability to take your body "for granted" this way, plus the twin peaks of focus and relaxation we've explored, are what allow athletes to play in The Zone. Combined, they are probably the biggest keys to peak performance.

So you can see that this mastery isn't a master/slave kinda thing, it's more like a martial arts or Zen mastery—you know, when archers don't even have to look at the target anymore, that kind of thing. You don't dominate and control your body to get it to perform. Instead, you rely on it confidently to perform and then release it, letting go of conscious control—and that's true power.

This phenomenon has been recognized in both yoga and the burgeoning field of sports science. In yoga, it's usually referred to as "harmony" between body and mind; in sports it's known as proprioceptive awareness. The term "proprioception" literally means a sense of the self. In this context it means the cumulative sense that we get, through all the information our body's sensors constantly feed us, about our environment and the appropriate reactions to it. Basically, proprioception tells us, in microseconds, what's going on and what to do about it. And in athletics especially, the more info you can get and process intuitively—this is a totally unconscious process—the better off you are.

"That enhanced proprioceptive awareness is something that all the great ones have, something that sets them apart," says Titans strength and conditioning coach Steve Watterson. "Part of it is the ability to adapt—to torn-up turf, say, to use an example from our sport. Another part is bi-hemisphere ability, when you can be doing completely different things with your upper and lower extremities—without thinking about either of them. I'm thinking of **Michael Jordan** and **Larry Bird** and some of the things they could do."

Speaking of Larry Legend: Another advantage he, Michael Jordan and other superstars like **Wayne Gretzky** were known for is their ability to see two or three moves ahead of everyone else. This not only helps them see plays develop but also protects against injury; if you anticipate contact and fall with awareness and control, you're less likely to get hurt. Yoga helps you develop this intuitive anticipation.

As Eric Paskel puts it: "'Intuition' is really heightened awareness." And we know that yoga fine-tunes your awareness.

Four years into his practice, goalie **Sean Burke** sees these kinds of changes in himself and his game. Let him tell it:

"Being an NHL goalie sometimes you're sore or hurt and it's almost like you don't want to have to subject yourself to all the pain and punishment that's coming up the ice every single shift. But I've noticed a big difference in that area. Now when there's scrambles in front of the net and bodies are flying all over the place, I don't worry about getting hurt or any of that.

"Plus, you have to be able to get up and get down incredibly quick, and I just have complete faith in my joints and ligaments. I know I can trust in my hips and groin and hamstrings, that my flexibility is such that I can withstand all that traffic and any contact. I don't have to think about it; I just seem to have more confidence than ever before.

"And *not* thinking about either of those things is huge in and of itself, because if your job is to focus on stopping pucks, you don't need anything else entering your mind while you're trying to do your job. One tiny little lapse can make all the difference in the world, and yoga has helped me understand that as much as anything."

Big-time yogis can get to this unconscious performance state in their game as well. Michael Lechonczak, our technical consultant on this book, has been practicing for 15 years and teaching for 10. At this point, he says, "I know what athletes are talking about when they talk about The Zone. When I'm doing yoga, I'm so deep into my practice and my body, I just never think 'I'm going to fall,' or anything like that. And in that deep, deep place, I absolutely own my body."

"It's not like my body is a *thing*, though," he continues. "Some people seem to relate to their bodies as if they were machines, like some Oldsmobiles that they drive around to get from here to there. But I'm just really grounded and present in my body, I'm witnessing my breath, my brain is connecting all the dots, and the practice just unfolds."

If you stick with your yoga training, you may first experience this flow state there. Or it may be while playing some sport you enjoy. Maybe you'll even experience peak performance in both! The point is, you're more likely to get in The Zone—and arrive there sooner and visit more often—because of the concentrated effort you've put in on the mat. I've just had a couple glimpses of it myself. It's pretty sweet, you'll see.

Twenty-first-century medicine is currently turning its attention to peak performance and how it can be instilled and improved. In elite athletic labs like the U.S. Olympic Training Center in Colorado, scientists think up ways to stimulate all the body's tiny sensors that send proprioceptive information to the brain. And they're finding out, as yoga teachers have long known, that the central nervous system can become more responsive in turning this information into instant actions.

You know what they do there? Lots of exercises for balance and stability. (You may have seen outgrowths of this in your gym, such as the Swiss ball and balance boards.) There's also frequent changes of body position, extending the customary range of motion, and twisting, rotational movements. Hmm . . . sound like any other exercise method you may have heard of recently?

There's even a new-wave approach to physical therapy called Proprioceptive Neuromuscular Facilitation (PNF). While other kinds of rehab isolate, focusing on one joint or one motion at a time, PNF uses natural overall patterns of movement that recruit many body parts. Again, sound familiar?

Cutting-edge Western medicine and the Eastern yoga tradition are two converging paths to the same destination: greater awareness, control and deep trust of your body, promoting peak performance. By beginning your yoga practice with this book you've already started on your way to reaching your ultimate athletic potential.

Next we're going to move on to another kind of peak performance, one that's also enhanced by yoga in amazing, synergistic ways. That's right, I'm talking about S-E-X. And we'll learn a new exercise that helps men play in The Zone there, too.

CHAPTER 16
Sex: The Yoga Bonus (For Both of You)

Guess what? No high-profile professional athletes wanted to go on the record and talk about their sex lives and yoga. In fact, no Real Men would be quoted by name, either. (Don't look at me; I have a wife, too, and she would not appreciate me going public with those details).

But I know you're curious. The dirty Downward Dog in you is wondering if all this enhanced flexibility and body awareness is going to pay off in the sack.

It is. To put it in guy terms, yoga and sex go together like Final and Four. I'm not talking about Tantric sex, which you may have heard celebrities like Sting going on about. Truth is, the Tantric tradition, a variant on both Buddhism and Hinduism that dates from around the sixth century, is really only about half of 1 percent about sex. And the part that's about sex is pretty far out there for most of us mainstream guys (especially the Tantric ideas about not ejaculating; what's up with that?). Let's just keep it to regular old twentieth-century American sex. That's plenty good enough—and, as you'll see, with yoga, it gets even better.

Take it from one guy interviewed for this book who just didn't want me to use his name. His report from the bedroom? "My wife really likes it when I am doing yoga, and she can definitely tell when I'm practicing more regularly," says Mr. Anonymous. "She'll say, 'You need to keep doing that.' I'm telling you, the effect is there."

Anonymous is only in his 30s and he feels a definite difference.

Older guys will appreciate yoga's Viagra-like effects even more.

How does yoga amp up your sex life? As usual, it works in many overlapping and simultaneous ways. Physically, the stretching sends greater blood flow through your muscles, and that stimulates all the nerve endings in there. That alone can make you feel more alive and thus more horny.

Yoga also gives you a boost in specific areas that matter for sex: the groin, hips and pelvis. The hip and groin openers, like the **Pigeon** and **Crescent Moon,** give you more elasticity and bounce "down there." The **Cat Stretch** is great at loosening up the pelvis, too. Naturally, guys with back pain—definitely not conducive to All-Star quality lovemaking—will also appreciate the improvements in their sex lives when yoga helps take that pain away.

Fatigue is a big sex-killer for men. Sometimes this can be just an excuse, the male equivalent of "Not tonight, honey, I have a headache." Often, though, it's real: We're just too worn out to get busy late at night. However, as several men have already testified, yoga energizes your entire body. You may not even need as much sleep when you're practicing.

Michael sums up the yoga-sex thing well: "When you do yoga, your body is happier. Your partner will also be happier."

It goes beyond the physical, though. Yoga gives you an additional boost on that psychological level—and you know that most of our sexual response really happens in the brain. So if you are using the "too-tired" thing as an excuse, doing yoga may improve your overall mood and outlook so much that you won't want to plead fatigue anymore.

For one thing, says L.A. instructor Jennifer Greenhut, "You feel more accepting of your body." I would take it a step further and say that as you get better at yoga, you aren't just accepting of your body, but really pleased with it, loving its newfound capabilities and wanting to explore its potential even further. That gets *you* going, plus it's a very short step from there to being able to appreciate *someone else's* body in the same way. And that can make for a very sexy situation. (For maximum results, you've gotta get your partner into yoga, too.)

Practicing helps you to be more present and focused, which obviously helps when you're trying to do the do. The last thing you or your partner need is for you to be distracted or somewhere else mentally. Mr. Anonymous thinks that's where yoga's done him the most good, sex-wise. "For my wife, I think it's my greater flexibility and range of motion," he says. "But for me, it's putting away distraction and being in the moment—not thinking about anything else, just letting go."

Stress is death on our sex lives, but yoga is the antidote. In the flight-or-fight reaction we have to stressors (we talked about this in chapter 13), blood flows to the extremities and away from the genital area. Makes sense from an evolutionary standpoint: there's no use getting all aroused while you're fighting or fleeing. And some believe that the inflammatory chemicals secreted when we're under stress—including modern-day psychological strain—can depress the reproductive system in the same way they're known to suppress the immune system. So that puts a cramp in the old libido.

Yoga lowers stress levels by damping the stress response of the sympathetic nervous system. In addition, it bolsters the parasympathetic system, the counterpart that regulates healing, sleep and digestion, and also promotes reproductive health. When this mellower, feel-good system is enhanced by yoga's fuller breathing, long stretches and deep relaxation, you get greater sexual vitality.

Makes sense, both common and medical. Though it might seem like the opposite is true, erection is a function of relaxation. When you get aroused, the muscles surrounding penile arteries relax, allowing the arteries to dilate (open) and allow more blood to flow into the penis. Viagra works by causing that dilation.

Yoga can also protect your sexual health. Anxiety and vascular problems are two main causes of impotence or erectile dysfunction (ED), and we know that yoga counteracts them both. Some yoga proponents take this even further. Traditional yoga teachers and believers think that the asanas don't just help your muscles and breathing, but also massage and invigorate the internal organs, including the prostate gland. It's their belief that exercises such as the **Cobra,** the **Bow,** the **Locust** and others help keep the prostate functioning optimally and even lessen the severity of prostate illness, including cancer.

All these important benefits for your sex life will come with regular yoga practice—a bonus or extra perk. However, for those guys seeking even more of an upgrade, as it were, here's a supplemental exercise that many yoga instructors and sex therapists believe will help both performance and long-term health.

Known as Kegel exercises, after the surgeon who popularized them in the United States back in the 1950s, it works the pubococcygeus, a complex of pelvic muscles that cradle the internal sexual organs, running from the pubic bone to the tailbone across the perineum, the area between the scrotum and the anus. Usually referred to as one "PC" muscle for simplicity's sake, or even "The Love Muscle," it contracts or spasms involuntarily during orgasm (women have it too). Flexing and strengthening the PC brings a greater blood supply, as with any other muscle, and is said to intensify sensation and help men delay and control ejaculation.

Interestingly enough, in the Kundalini tradition, the perineum is where energy supposedly enters the body. The more energy you take in there, it's believed, the hornier you get (I'm paraphrasing here). The Kegel is roughly equivalent to yoga's "mula bandha," a technique for locking in breath (or *prana*). Once again, East and West seem to converge and agree here.

So try a few Kegels—I'm calling them **Sex Squeezes,** because of the way this exercise operates—and see if you (and your partner) feel a difference. Isn't it about time you got in touch with your pubococcygeus, anyway?

SEX SQUEEZES

◆ Sit comfortably on a chair or on your mat.

◆ Breathe slowly and deeply. As you exhale, contract the PC muscles of the perineum, using the action you would use to stop the flow of urine. Or you can visualize the contraction drawing your testicles back toward the anus. Just take 1 or 2 seconds for the contraction, squeezing but not straining, then release.

◆ Repeat about 10 times at first and work up to 25 reps, performed twice daily. You can also gradually increase the duration, holding the contraction 2 to 3 seconds more, for about 5 seconds total.

◆ Please, do this slowly and gently and build up gradually. This ain't no bench press; the muscles involved are small and they will only get so strong. So don't overdo it, guys. You know that in this area of the body, pain is definitely not gain.

CHAPTER 17
Making It Work:
Yoga in Your Life

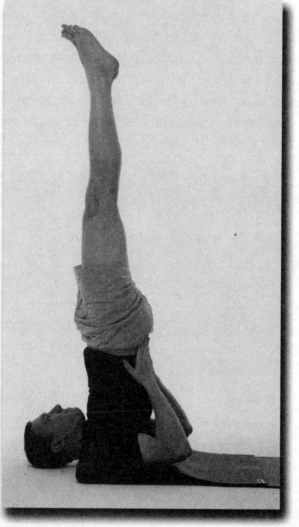

©Erica Berger, 2003

After you master all the yoga moves in this book, you can move on to trickier ones like the Shoulder Stand.

Okay, now you know it all. Or at least, you know everything you need to begin your yoga practice and start enjoying all these great benefits I've been going on about.

To do that, start using the workouts that follow this chapter. After you've done them for a while, I also recommend that you go to some yoga classes. That may sound strange coming from a guy who's written a yoga book, but I'm really just trying to get you started, to give you a foundation. After you use this book you can go ahead and get some in-person instruction and continue to move forward in your practice. You need feedback on your posture and movement, plus you can learn the trickier positions I've omitted here, such as the **Shoulder Stand** (previous page), **Headstand** and **Handstand** (below).

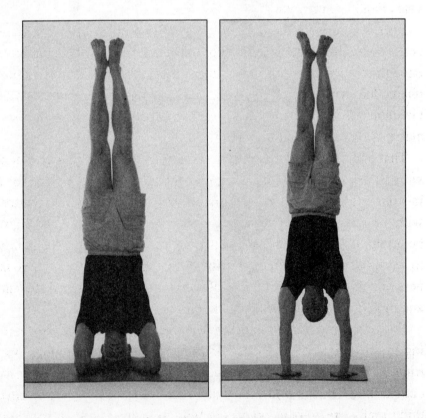

Doing the work and learning the exercises in the book first also eliminates one big reason lots of guys don't go to yoga classes: We don't want to be ignorant and embarrassed, the only dummy in the room who doesn't know what's going on. (For some of us, this is worse than asking directions while driving!) Now you're up to speed, ready to roll into any class with confidence.

You probably won't be the only guy in the class, either. That's changing rapidly these days as more and more men get into yoga. In fact, Hilary Lindsay, who works with running back **Eddie George** down in Nashville, teaches a 6:30 A.M. class on Tuesdays and Thursdays. "It's almost all guys," she says. "A lot of 'em are in real estate, they're businessmen and entrepreneurs—and most of my private clients are men, too."

Even if you were the only guy, would that be so bad? You'll get crazy points from the women there for being open-minded and brave enough to show up. And, of course, there's the visuals, the atmosphere, the surround, if you will. As L.A. yoga instructor Jennifer Greenhut says, "There's a lot of girls with cute yoga butts in those classes." (Hey, she said it, not me!)

That could be a good incentive for hitting classes regularly. But as with all exercise programs, it's a real challenge to find a place for it in your life and develop a consistent yoga routine. Mixing classes with your own private workouts gives you some variety and fights boredom. I also urge you to find a yoga buddy, like a running buddy, to work out and/or go to class with. This can minimize any nervousness you might feel about trying classes with more advanced students and motivate both buddies to stick with their practices.

Try your wife or girlfriend as your yoga buddy. I'll bet she's willing to do some with you. Men and women often have a tough time running or strength-training together, but they're completely yoga-compatible. Though you really do yoga by yourself, there's something really great about practicing with your loved one in the same room. This can really turn into "quality time" for the two of you.

Discover the virtues of "yoga to go." By that I mean that yoga is so portable, it's great for guys who travel a lot on business. Glen de Vries, our model in all the book's yoga photos, is 31 and the chief technology officer for Medidata Solutions. He goes to classes about 2 to 4 times in an average week, but he's on the road a lot, often making one-day trips from his New York base to the West Coast. "Rather than have to pack sneakers and sweat stuff and then try to deal with some broken treadmill in a hotel gym," Glen says, "I do my own yoga workout in the room. If I have an hour, I'll turn down the lights and do a full routine, with breathing exercises, inversions and everything. Or sometimes I'll just do 10 minutes in the morning while watching CNN."

Glen's made a commitment to yoga and he's keeping it. He also swims, lifts, runs some, and he's thinking about triathlons. So he's a prime example of using yoga as cross-training. This fact should inspire you, as you look at him nailing all the poses in these pictures: He's only been doing yoga for two years.

Now it's your turn. It's up to you to do the work like a Real Man should. Yoga's well worth it, I promise you. In fact, if you have any questions or comments about yoga or this book, I encourage you to e-mail me at *johnc@realmendoyoga.com,* and I'll be glad to help you out in any way I can. For now, I'll just encourage you to begin your yoga practice, and I sincerely hope that you end up loving it as much as I do. You've probably heard that old saying about the road (to somewhere, I forget where exactly) beginning with a single step. I'd like to paraphrase that with yoga in mind, and close by saying this: The road to greater health and happiness begins with a single stretch.

CHAPTER 18

Get with the Program! Yoga Workouts for Rookies & Veterans

These two routines cover all the bases: generating some heat; promoting proper alignment; developing flexibility, strength and balance; integrating back bends, forward folds and spinal twists. I asked Michael Lechonczak, the master yoga teacher we've heard from throughout the book, to devise them with guys in mind. The sequencing is very important, so please do them in order.

Do the first one, a 30-minute routine for rookies or beginners, twice a week for 6 to 8 weeks, or until you're doing all the exercises without much strain and with good form. This list of positions will refer you back to the pages with complete instructions (and bigger pictures) to follow. For at least the first month or so, stick to the standard ways of doing the poses, leaving the Super-Charge It variations for later. Some poses will come hard; others, easy. It's that way for everyone.

Three workouts a week would be even better. I know you're a busy guy, but three times will increase your benefits exponentially.

Then you can graduate to the veterans workout, a tougher sequence that will take about 45 minutes. Try hard to keep your number of workouts a week up, even though that means more time. Go ahead and add in the Super-Charged variations if you like, but be careful, as with all the moves, not to go too hard too fast. Remember, there's no such sport as competitive yoga. So there's no need to try to outdo anyone—even yourself. If you feel like you are struggling, or just want a change of pace, it's fine to go back to the first workout.

After you've done the veterans workout for 2 to 3 months, you should be pretty proficient, but still feel yourself making progress—getting more flexible and deeper into poses, gaining greater control over your breathing. At this point, you can begin to hold the positions longer (say, half again as many breaths) to up the intensity.

After that, you're on your own. Just keep going and you'll have a terrific practice. Or, as I suggested in the last chapter, take your new yoga act public and hit some classes. You can learn and improve infinitely. And enjoy. Real Man Yoga is supposed to be fun yoga, so keep approaching it that way—and you'll keep doing it.

ROOKIES WORKOUT

30 minutes

Note: Do all poses one time, unless otherwise noted.

Three-Part Breath (page 79).

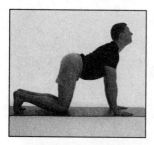

Cat Stretch (page 19).

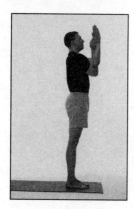

Half Eagle (page 20).

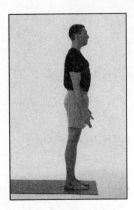

Sun Salutes (page 101). Three full reps; that is, do the sequence 6 times, alternately leading with each foot 3 times.

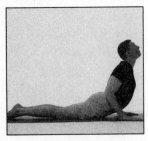

Front Plank (page 53).

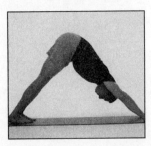

Cobra (page 12).

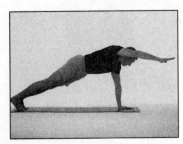

Downward Dog (page 35).

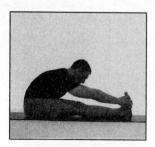

Seated Forward Bend (page 117).

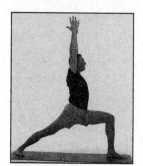

Warrior I (page 49). Two reps, one with each foot leading.

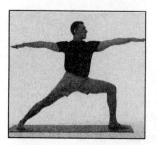

Warrior II (page 50).

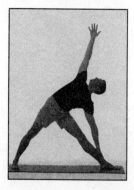

Triangle (page 90).

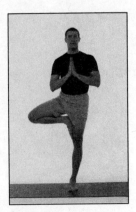

Tree (page 65).

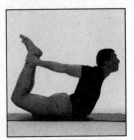

Bow (page 22).

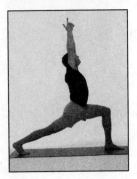

Crescent Moon (page 37). Remember to do it with the knee down first.

Pigeon Alternate (page 42).

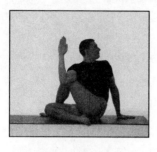

Seated Twist (page 24).

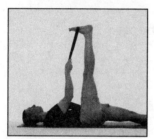

Hamstring Stretch (page 34).

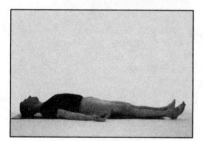

5-Minute Relaxation (page 145).

Optional:

Toe Balance (page 138), for extra balance/focus work. Insert after **Tree.**

Breath Awareness Meditation (page 152), for greater focus and deeper relaxation. Do after relaxation at end of workout or any time.

Sex Squeezes (page 173). Add to end of workout or do any time.

VETERANS WORKOUT

45 minutes

Note: Do all poses one time, unless otherwise noted.

Three-Part Breath (page 79).

Power Exhales (page 81).

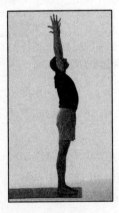

Sun Salutes (page 101). Three full reps.

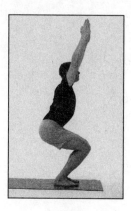

Chair (page 51).

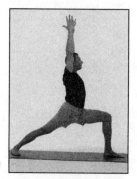

Warrior I (page 49).

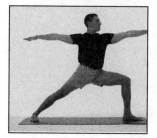

Warrior II (page 50).

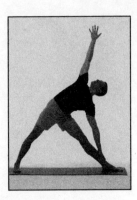

Triangle (page 90).

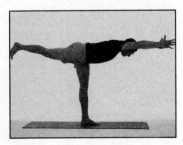

Warrior III (page 71).

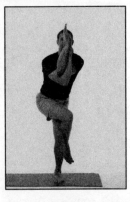

Eagle (page 68).

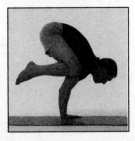

Crow (page 69).

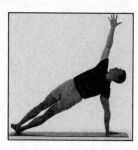

Side Plank (page 54).

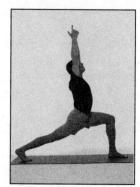

Crescent Moon (page 37). With knee down.

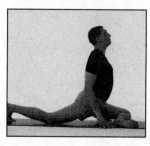

Pigeon (page 40).

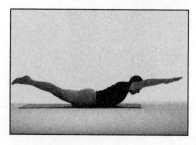

Half Locust (page 93) and **Full Locust** (shown) (page 94).

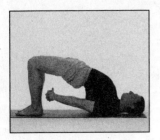

Bridge (page 118).

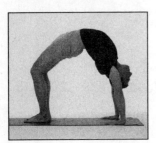

Wheel (page 57).

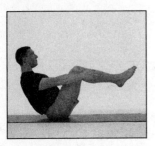

Boat, Half (page 92) (shown) or **Full** (page 93).

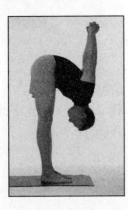

Arms-Up Forward Bend (page 126).

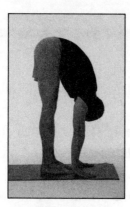

Standing Forward Bend
(page 115).

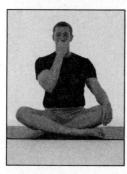

Kneeling Twist (page 25).

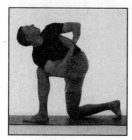

Alternate Nostril Breathing
(page 84).

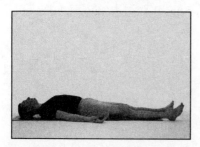

5-Minute Relaxation (page 145).

___

Optional:

Toe Balance (page 138), for extra balance/focus work. Insert after **Crow.**

Breath Awareness Meditation (page 152), for greater focus and deeper relaxation. Do after **5-Minute Relaxation** at end of workout or any time.

Sex Squeezes (page 173). Add to end of workout or do any time.

___

About the Author

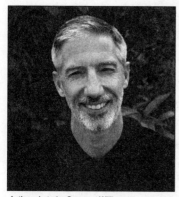

Author photo by Suzanne Williamson

A journalist, sportswriter and a yoga practitioner, **John Capouya** is currently the deputy editor of *SmartMoney* magazine. He was formerly the health and medicine editor of *Newsweek,* a features editor at *The New York Times* and the editor of *Pro,* the magazine for professional athletes. His sports writing has been anthologized in *The Best Sports Stories* book series, and he is a graduate of Grinnell College and the Columbia University Graduate School of Journalism. Capouya lives in New York City with his wife, photographer and photo editor Suzanne Williamson. He practices at the Dharma Yoga Center in New York City and with Michael Lechonczak.

About the Contributors

Michael Lechonczak, consultant and advisor on *Real Men Do Yoga,* has been practicing and teaching yoga for more than 15 years. Trained extensively in the Iyengar, Ashtanga and Anusara approaches to Hatha yoga, Michael sees private clients in New York City and also teaches exclusively at the Equinox Fitness clubs there. With his wife, Robin, he leads yoga retreats internationally, and will soon be launching a series of Real Man retreats. Michael can be contacted at *nyyogaman@nyc.rr.com.* His upcoming book is entitled *Real People, Real Yoga.*

Erica Berger, who photographed the yoga poses for this book, has shot for *Time, Newsweek, People, Life, Forbes* and the *Washingtonian,* among other clients. Her work can be licensed through the Corbis/Outline agency and can be seen at *ericaberger.com.*

Glen de Vries, who demonstrates all the yoga poses, is the chief technology officer for Medidata Solutions, a clinical research software company based in New York City. He has been studying yoga with Michael Lechonczak for just over two years.

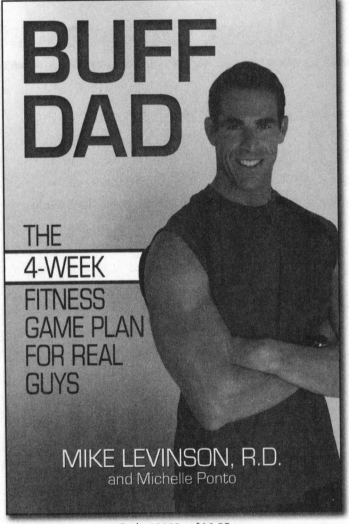

BUFF DAD

THE 4-WEEK FITNESS GAME PLAN FOR REAL GUYS

MIKE LEVINSON, R.D.
and Michelle Ponto

Code #6160 • $16.95

Begin the program that delivers motivational tips,
exercise guidelines, and diet advice to burn off pounds
without burning away precious time.